Ray Ridolfi was born in Australia, and first became interested in Oriental medicine whilst studying law and the arts in Brisbane.

Ray Ridolfi has worked in the bodywork field for 14 years and is co-founder and Principal of the British School of Shiatsu-Do which is based at the East West Centre in London. He is also a senior member of the Shiatsu Society, sitting on the Practitioner Assessment Panel and on the Ethics Committee. He has written numerous articles on shiatsu and has taught extensively in Europe and the Middle East. This is his first book.

ALTERNATIVE HEALTH

SHIATSU

RAY RIDOLFI

ILLUSTRATED BY SHAUN WILLIAMS

An OPTIMA book

First published in 1990 by
Macdonald Optima, a division of
Macdonald & Co. (Publishers) Ltd

Reprinted 1990

A member of Maxwell Macmillan Pergamon Publishing Corporation

British Library Cataloguing in Publication Data
Ridolfi, Ray
  Shiatsu.
  1. Shiatsu
  I. Title   II. Series
  615.8'22

  ISBN 0-356-17181-7

Macdonald & Co (Publishers) Ltd
Orbit House
1 New Fetter Lane
London EC4A 1AR

Typeset by Leaper & Gard Ltd, Bristol
Printed and bound in Great Britain by
The Guernsey Press Co. Ltd, Guernsey, Channel Islands

Dedication

To my wife, Jill for all her support. Special thanks to my shiatsu teacher, colleague and friend Saul Goodman and to Wataru Ohashi *sensei* for his guidance.

Contents

PREFACE

For centuries, people have sought effective ways in which to help one another in times of need. The medium of touch serves this purpose well. Touch has different applications, such as in cases of fear, anger, love, sympathy, compassion, or desire. The intention behind this action is the important determining factor of the effect of the touch sensation.

For many years I have been interested in health and exercise. I was always considered to be the 'health fanatic' by my friends. It still amuses me to consider the thinking behind such sayings. Being conscious of one's health seems to be an unnatural occurrence in modern society. This initial interest in my own health led me to look at the health of others around me. Being very active in sport, I found that I was very successful at injuring myself. This of course gave me the opportunity to research sports injury medicine to heal myself. Here began my real interest in the physical body and its functioning.

Eventually I came to realise that my consciousness and ability to maintain a happy frame of mind greatly depended on my physical condition. The fitter I became, the better my concentration at work and leisure. I was studying to be a solicitor in Australia at the time and my examination and work results also seemed to reflect my condition. Subsequently, as a solicitor, I found myself working in matrimonial law. The sorrow and stress of divorce clients suffering the trauma of separation from children and partners often created frustration for me. These people needed to be held and comforted and ethically I couldn't do this.

On reflection, I now understand that I could have helped these people more effectively with shiatsu than verbal advice. Sure, they needed technical, legal advice but what they required emotionally was compassionate understanding given without reservation or attachments.

This is shiatsu. I find it amusing that these days I am often treating lawyers for stress as well as people with relationship problems.

Shiatsu has a much wider effect than most people think. Anyone working with shiatsu appreciates the emotional and psychological strengthening that often occurs in the course of regular shiatsu treatments. This change also has a much deeper effect on the individual's consciousness and understanding of their place in our environment and society. It's what the Buddhists call 'Big Mind' – a state of mind where the individual becomes aware of his or her place in the 'whole' of society and how each action of the individual, no matter how small, affects the 'whole'. If everyone in the world became more conscious of this relationship it would be a healthier and happier place. For me, shiatsu takes us all a little closer to this ideal.

Ray Ridolfi
London 1989

1
SHIATSU THERAPY: ORIGIN AND USAGE

WHAT IS SHIATSU?

Shiatsu is a Japanese word, translating literally as 'finger pressure'. A wider translation is 'to apply pressure to the body using the fingers'. Shiatsu is sometimes referred to in the West as acupressure. The application of pressure to the body surface is the underlying principle of shiatsu; the therapist will not only use fingers to apply pressure, but the use of palms, elbows, feet and knees is also common practice. The thumb is the most important tool of the therapist.

Touch is our most essential form of communication. Touch may be loving or aggressive, intuitive or mechanical; touch is a therapy in itself. The healing benefits of this communication medium are experienced every day. A child's bruised knee is 'healed' by a loving parental caress; a moment of sadness is relieved by the supporting hug of a friend. It is the feeling behind the offered touch which makes all the difference.

Shiatsu therapy works on the principle that touching in a caring manner helps trigger self-healing in the patient. Everyone experiences a 'need' to be touched in some form, and the shiatsu therapist aims to fulfil this need. Shiatsu is primarily preventative, in that it can be used to maintain good health as well as help improve poor health, resulting in a heightened sense of well-being.

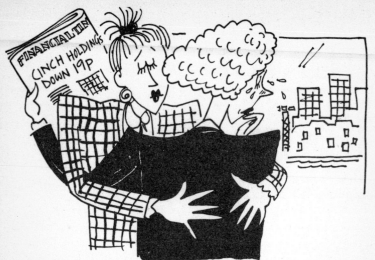

... A MOMENT OF SADNESS IS RELIEVED BY THE SUPPORTING HUG OF A FRIEND ...

THE ENERGY SYSTEM

Shiatsu acts on the subtle electromagnetic energy of the body, described as *ki* in Japanese and *chi* in Chinese. The ancient Chinese exercise called *tai chi* stimulates the movement of *chi*. In Oriental medicine, *ki* is considered as our life 'essence' which maintains and nurtures our physical body and therefore affects also the mind and spirit. The human body cannot be separated into individual parts functioning separately to one another: our physical body is a field of continually moving energy, circulating through the cells, tissues, muscles and organs.

Ki flows through all the organs and body areas through a system of channels or pathways known as meridians. These meridians are like an efficient irrigation system, ensuring the nurturing of all bodily functions when energy is flowing unimpaired. Along these meridians are high electromagnetically charged areas or pressure points known as *tsubo* in Japanese. Stimulation of the *tsubo* affects the flow of *ki* along the meridians as well as other areas of the body. There are twelve major meridians containing in excess of 700 *tsubo* throughout the energy system.

Each meridian supplies energy to a specific organ or system in the body. As in an irrigation system, should a meridian or *tsubo* become blocked the area and bodily functions nurtured by this meridian will enter a state of dis-ease, a condition of stress. We all wish to achieve a state of 'ease' and the release of blocked *ki* in a meridian or body area helps to achieve this healthier and more 'balanced' condition. The shiatsu therapist uses different techniques to release energy blockages, including stretching, rubbing, corrective exercises, together with the primary use of finger pressure to 'open' the meridians.

THE HISTORY OF SHIATSU

As with Western medicine, Oriental medicine developed out of a need to maintain good health and prevent illness. Oriental medical philosophy in China developed over a 3,000 to 5,000 year period and is often difficult to understand using a Western scientific clinical approach. The natural growth of Oriental medicine is based on thousands of years of trial-and-error experimentation in practice.

The main forms of traditional Oriental medical therapy are massage (known as *amma*), acupuncture, moxibustion (the burning of a herb, moxa, on *tsubo*) and herbalism. Geographical, religious and philosophical factors determined the type of therapy developed in a particular area of China. Geographically, China is divided by the Yangtze (Yellow) River and in the past the medical approaches were divided into the northern and southern branches. South of the Yangtze were fertile lands where the growth and usage of herbs and tree barks to prepare medicinal remedies flourished. The more barren, rocky lands in the north were less suitable to herb growth and here the people relied on the physical therapies of massage and moxa. Through the experimentation with massage and the development of the theory of the

meridian system, the additional therapy of acupuncture
evolved.

Amma was used extensively as a helpful remedy for
common ailments. It is a technique of rubbing and
pressing the body, and became very popular in the Edo
period (1501–1857), subsequently establishing itself in
Japan through both the trading and warring which went
on between China and Japan. This type of therapy
developed in the same manner as Western massage, which
had its birthplace in France. As early as the fourth and
fifth centuries BC written records of the era show that
Hippocrates promoted the use of massage. Other founding
fathers of Western medicine such as Herophilus and
Erasistratus (Alexandria, third century) theorised about
the energy system. They thought that nerves were hollow
pathways transmitting 'vital spirit' – interestingly close to
Oriental medical theory.

In Japan, *amma* (known as *anma* in Japanese) was
practised mainly by blind therapists, who were
supposedly more sensitive than their sighted colleagues;
because the loss of the sense of sight, the sense of touch
becomes pronounced. This form of massage differed
greatly from Western massage in one major area –
diagnosis. The ability to diagnose a problem and design a
specific treatment accordingly made this therapy unique
at that time. This massage system eventually became
known as shiatsu. Early this century, shiatsu therapists
incorporated many Western techniques such as those
used in chiropractic and osteopathy. Today, shiatsu is
continually being improved, as are Western medical
techniques, and research into its effects in both the East
and West has made it a well respected therapy.

COULD SHIATSU HELP ME?

In 1955 shiatsu was given official recognition in Japan.
The Japanese Ministry of Health and Welfare stated that
'Shiatsu therapy is a form of manipulation administered
by the thumbs, fingers and palms, without the use of any

instrument, mechanical or otherwise, to apply pressure to the human skin, correct internal malfunctioning, promote and maintain health, and treat specific diseases.'

The combination of diagnostic and treatment techniques involving stretching, corrective exercises and pressure application helps promote an improved physical and emotional condition. Shiatsu can remove physical stiffness and pain, increase mobility and flexibility of limbs and joints, improve circulation and toxic elimination, tone up the skin, strengthen the bones, improve the immune system, strengthen the muscles, as well as help to eliminate fatigue and stress.

THE EFFECTS OF SHIATSU

Shiatsu affects the receiver at the different levels of body, mind and spirit. The energy system is the primary concern of the therapist, who must try not to separate these different levels of health. It is important not to break down the patient's condition into a series of separate symptoms all requiring the attention of different specialists, such as is often the case in allopathic medicine.

The shiatsu therapist therefore takes a holistic view of the patient and determines all the factors involved. In this way, each treatment will be tailored to the specific needs of the patient. Everyone is an individual with a wealth of differing experiences and backgrounds, leading to either good health or poor health. For example, a migraine headache sufferer will describe a number of different causes potentially responsible for their condition. These may be muscular or skeletal injury, nervous tension, menstrual problems, digestive problems, environmental factors such as noise, central heating, air-conditioning, family or work stress – the list goes on, depending on the individual's background. If ten people all suffer from migraines there may be innumerable and drastically differing causes in each case. A pain relief drug designed to suppress the symptoms of migraine will obviously be

SHIATSU CAN HELP:

- Relieve stress and tension.

- Calm the nervous system.

- Stabilise emotional and psychological conditions.

- Improve digestion.

- Improve libido.

- Relieve menstrual problems.

- Ease childbirth.

- Ease sports injuries.

- Relieve backache.

- Strengthen body, mind and spirit.

- Improve stamina.

- Relief aches and pains.

- Relieve headaches.

- Improve vitality and general health.

- Promote healthy pregnancy.

- Create body awareness.

- Help prevent common illnesses.

- Improve posture.

inadequate in most cases, as is proved time and time again. The treatment must be more personal than this, and based on all the historical factors of the patient. In fact every shiatsu treatment is unique for this reason.

Physical effects

The skin   The human skin acts as our physical protective layer. The skin breathes – it is considered part of our respiratory system – and is a reflection of our internal condition. The body's ability to detoxify itself and eliminate waste products effectively can also be seen by the condition of the skin. Lung meridian energy predominantly controls the skin function, but other organ energies will always be involved, behind the scenes so to speak; for example, the heart constrictor and triple warmer will control the *ki* and blood supply to feed the lubricating system for the skin.

The sweat glands as well as the sebaceous glands moisturise and give nutrition to the skin. The sweat glands rid the body of wastes such as carbon dioxide, and impaired stimulation of these glands causes fatigue due to the retention of excess carbon dioxide. If more than a third of the total skin surface is damaged, as in burn cases, death may occur. Shiatsu will help stimulate circulation to the skin, activating the capillaries in the skin tissue, the dermal cells and the sebaceous glands, thus aiding the secretion of essential body oils and keeping the skin moist, smooth and in good tune.

Muscular system   The muscles are responsible for locomotion. Muscles are connected to the bones and joints, for example enabling you to bend your elbow or leg, or hold this book. All of your muscles are tensed throughout your waking hours, even when sitting or in other states of apparent inactivity. They only completely relax when you sleep. This is the time when rejuvenation should be occurring.

Liver meridian energy predominantly controls the muscles. If there is stress and muscular tension, particularly upon wakening, the muscle fibres may be stiffening due to stagnation of energy hindering the circulation of blood and lymph. Muscles need to be nourished with energy to maintain a healthy toned condition. Pressure to the skin surface penetrates to the muscles, stimulating the movement of *ki*, blood and lymph and thus making the muscle fibres thicken, strengthening the joints.

Skeletal system   The primary function of the skeletal system is protection; the bones of the cranium protect the brain, the ribs protect the heart, lungs and abdominal organs, the pelvic girdle protects the lower digestive and reproductive organs. The combined function of the

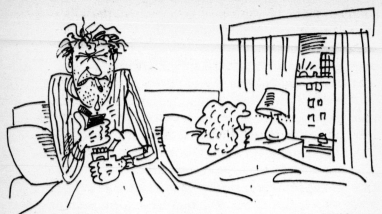

... IF THERE IS STRESS AND MUSCULAR TENSION, PARTICULARLY UPON AWAKENING, THE MUSCLE FIBRES MAY BE STIFFENING DUE TO STAGNATION OF ENERGY HINDERING THE CIRCULATION OF BLOOD AND LYMPH....

muscles and bones give us the locomotion system referred to above.

The body is made up of 70 per cent water, and the bones themselves are 80 per cent water. It is for this reason that the kidney meridian energy which controls water metabolism also controls bone quality. Shiatsu will help stimulate the circulation and flow of important nutrients which maintain and strengthen the bones and joints.

Circulatory system   The heart is the central organ of this system. Blood is pumped to all parts of the body through the arteries and returns to the heart in the venous system. The condition of the heart, arteries and veins can be weakened greatly by lack of exercise and poor diet; circulation to the extremities is often impaired, varicose veins appear and swelling of the extremities may occur. All these problems may be alleviated by improving the condition of the heart and its capability of pumping healthy blood around the body.

The heart and heart governor meridians control circulation. Shiatsu will aid the movement of blood and help strengthen a weakened venous and arterial system, although exercise and an improved diet is also necessary, of course.

Nervous system　The nervous system is responsible for the transmission of information to all parts of the body. Messages travel from the brain to stimulate the muscles in your hands, for example 'instructing' them to perform functions as required. Pain messages are referred back to the brain to allow the body to react to danger.

The nerves control the bodily functions through the central and autonomic nervous systems. The central system consists of the spinal cord, inside the spinal vertebrae, and the cerebrum in the head. We are able to control this system consciously via the brain, whereas the autonomic nervous system is concerned with reflex control of bodily functions and cannot be controlled at will.

If your energy systems are sluggish and the time taken to react to danger or other everyday situations is slow, then life may be uncomfortable, with symptoms such as cramps, sprains, pulled muscles and torn tendons. The bladder meridian energy controls the nervous function; regular shiatsu and exercise will help keep the nerves alert.

Alimentary system　This is the digestive system, and is responsible for the intake of nourishment, and consequently fresh energy, to fuel all the bodily functions. The intake and assimilation of food sustains a nutritional balance and determines the amount and quality of energy available to you. Several meridian energies control this system, namely the large intestine, stomach and liver.

Waste deposits may accumulate in the digestive system unless you choose your food well and chew very conscientiously. A general lack of fitness will also be reflected in this system, causing complaints such as constipation, diarrhoea and ulcers. Shiatsu will aid the stimulation of digestive juice and enzymes.

Endocrine and exocrine systems　These are respectively the ductless and ducted glandular systems of the body. The endocrine system is responsible for the internal secretion of hormones into the blood stream preserving the body's chemical balance. Examples of this type of gland are the pituitary, adrenal, and gonad functions. If this function is impaired, such problems as menstrual difficulties, skin eruptions, growth abnormalities, and erratic sexual libido may arise. The kidney meridian energy is the main influence on this system, whilst the gallbladder energy has a secondary role.

The exocrine glands are responsible for secretions to the external surface of the body. Examples of these are the sweat, mammary, and lacrimal glands: also the glands of the mouth and alimentary tract. The alimentary tract, although it runs internally in the body, is thought of as an extension of the external skin surface and is still a boundary between the external environment and the internal environment. This system may be influenced by both internal and external changes. Temperature and activity will affect the sweat glands, and chewing, as well as visual stimulation, affects the salivary glands.

The salivary glands are influenced by hunger. This has several interpretations. It may be hunger for physical or spiritual foods. Our hunger for acquiring material possessions and knowledge stimulates the body in different ways. The stomach meridian energy controls this wider aspect of hunger. An executive, hungry to climb the ladder of success, has strong self-image and determination, and will usually have an excess stomach energy condition. It is well known that people tend to salivate at times of visual excitement. This may be looking at food or perhaps at someone who they find sexually stimulating. Oriental philosophy considers that the stimulation of saliva production through chewing indirectly affects the stomach meridian energy, which in turn has a strong influence on the reproductive system. The acid/alkaline balance of the saliva is a reflection of the yin/yang balance of the metabolism. Shiatsu has a direct effect on this yin/yang balance.

As you can see a general shiatsu treatment will not only

act as a tonic and release blockages in the meridian system, it will also greatly improve the function of the entire metabolism.

Emotional and psychological effects

'How are you today?', you are often asked. Do you unreservedly reply 'Very good, thank you,' or do you qualify your reply, such as, 'Not too bad and not too good'? These different replies or attitudes display a wealth of information about your state of mental and emotional health. Everyone wants to be happy in life, a very simple and understandable desire. How we achieve this happiness is where we begin to have difficulties. Modern society places great emphasis on 'doing' things to achieve happiness. How often have you thought 'I was really happy when I was doing this or that.'

Many traditional philosophies promote the exact opposite of this method of seeking happiness. Buddhism, for example, promotes the experience of happiness through doing nothing, that is through meditation – sitting quietly still without any material aids to stimulate the senses, just enjoying the calmness of the moment. Many large multinational corporations have now seen the power of meditation and exercise to control stress and improve the work capabilities of their employees.

Unlike Western medicine, which gives particular focus to the anatomical, physiological and mental functions of people as separate entities, Oriental medical philosophy looks a stage beyond these physical realms, at the energetic body. In shiatsu there is an underlying principle that there is first the energy of life or lifeforce, which precedes the creation of the structure. The human body is simply a vessel containing this lifeforce. During the embryonic phase, this lifeforce condenses and expands at different rates, creating the various organs and body systems. Because our structure is made up of energy, if we can learn to manipulate this energy then the structure and all its different functions will also change in due course.

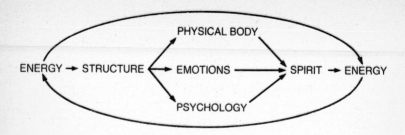

Think of the sequence in this diagram. This is a continuum of movement, and separation of the different levels of our being neglects the whole. There needs to be an intention of unification and not of separation of all aspects of ourselves. The common factor at all these levels is the influence of the life energy, and in shiatsu we therefore deal primarily with this.

Emotional and psychological changes are manifestations of energy movement. We all have felt the intimidating power of someone projecting their anger or frustration at us. How many times have you thought about telephoning someone, and they call you? This telepathic transference of energy is common; you can actually 'think' energy to someone and receive a response. By working on a patient's meridian system, the shiatsu therapist can see the energy blockages causing some particular emotional or psychological condition and treat it accordingly by unifying and unblocking the whole energy system.

We are all subject to stress, although some people seem to be able to cope and deal with stress more successfully than others. A major physiological factor here is the balance between the respective functions of the autonomic nervous system. This is divided into the sympathetic and parasympathetic systems, each having specific functions. Some of those functions affect breathing and heart rates, which change dramatically in times of stress or excitement. Shiatsu will assist the patient achieve what is commonly called the alpha state of relaxation, a subconscious state in which the parasympathetic mode of function is predominant. We all achieve this alpha state twice daily. Firstly when we begin to doze, sinking into deeper sleep, we enter a grey period of the alpha time – we are semiconscious and aware of our surroundings but calm and relaxed. We then go through the alpha state again as we change from deep sleep to full consciousness in the morning.

During a shiatsu treatment, the effect of this deep alpha relaxation allows the energy distortions affecting your emotions and mental condition to rebalance. Many a patient has exhibited a euphoric experience for a short time after the treatment as their energy settles.

QUESTIONS AND ANSWERS

How does shiatsu differ from acupuncture?
Both therapies work on the same basic principles of the 'wholeness' of the patient and the diagnosis of the energy system. Of course, a major difference is the use of needles in acupuncture. Some people have an aversion to needles and for them this may be enough reason to use shiatsu instead. I personally feel that shiatsu offers more of the nurturing aspect of therapy because of the direct contact during treatment. Remember that this is the basic comforting mechanism in our lives and for this reason shiatsu is very powerful in dealing with emotional and psychological conditions, when the patient is desperately wanting some physical attention which may be lacking in their daily life.

Another area of difference is the diagnostic methods used, as shiatsu places greater emphasis on the postural or body language and body diagnostic areas of the patient (see Chapter 4 for more details of diagnosis).

Acupuncture deserves no criticism and I regularly recommend my patients to try it in certain circumstances.

Is it different to massage?
Shiatsu is not considered to be massage in the common sense of the word. Massage, which takes many forms, can be powerful and is always helpful. Massage is primarily

for relaxation and leisure, although remedial massage is used to improve the circulation and lymph systems of the patient, thereby relieving many conditions of fatigue, muscular pain and general stress. The use of essential oils in aromatherapy is very beneficial for the relief of a large variety of problems.

However, the use of the many forms of diagnosis in shiatsu, based on thousands of years of clinical studies, allows the therapist to treat specific problems in a variety of ways. This may involve a different treatment every time you see your therapist, whereas in massage the same techniques are generally used on everyone. The treatment may also include the use of moxibustion, the burning of a herb on the *tsubo* to stimulate circulation and speed recovery, or the application of a particular compress or poultice.

Do I have to be ill to have shiatsu?

In ancient China and later in Japan, shiatsu or other therapies were originally used by certain gifted members of the family to help others, not only in times of injury or illness, but as a means of maintaining good health. Without their strength and stamina, rural people could not work the fields and therefore would go hungry. Much of the population of both countries was in the military, and shiatsu techniques were used to relax and strengthen the soldiers before battle and to revitalise them afterwards, as well as speeding the healing of their wounds. In the West we only go to see the doctor when we are ill; in the East the doctor was seen regularly and was dismissed as a failure if the patient ever became ill. The whole emphasis was on prevention and not cure.

You don't have to be ill to experience the benefits of shiatsu. If you simply wish to control your stress, feel calmer, have more patience, improve your stamina and powers of concentration, then shiatsu is for you. Think of it as an insurance policy against poor health. Most people mistakenly 'put off' doing maintenance exercises or dietary changes for the future in the belief that another

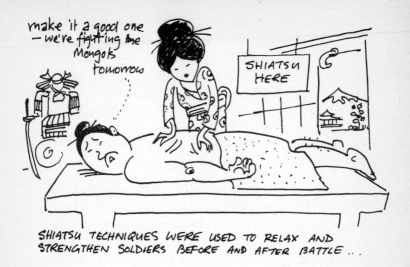

SHIATSU TECHNIQUES WERE USED TO RELAX AND
STRENGTHEN SOLDIERS BEFORE AND AFTER BATTLE...

day's delay won't matter. This delay inevitably extends
from days to months to years, until you are deeply
shocked into change by some overt change such as a
stroke or other major disorder.

If you wish to improve the quality of your life and
ensure longevity, you have to start now. Don't think 'It's
no use for me. I've already done too much damage so
what's the use of changing now?' Numerous elderly
patients I've treated who simply assumed they wouldn't
ever be able to enjoy gardening or walking any more, have
felt a new lease of life when their nagging backache or
arthritic pains have decreased. Conversely, many top
athletes, dancers, footballers and gymnasts have shiatsu
to maintain and improve their performances.

You can't buy good health; it takes a certain amount of
work and this of course means you have to take
responsibility for your own health and stop depending on
others. This theme of developing self responsibility
separates shiatsu from allopathic medicine and numerous
other therapies. Your shiatsu therapist will advise you on
exercise and diet to suit your needs. Indeed you are
expected to do more work than the therapist in your
journey to better health. You can consider the therapist as

an educator, whose job it is to help you rediscover your self-awareness and innate knowledge of self-health which most of us have forgotten because of the seemingly magical advances in modern medicine which have unfortunately taken away our need for self-responsibility. But don't despair; as a well known Taoist philosopher called Lao Tsu once said: 'The journey of a thousand miles starts with the first step.'

Are there people who shouldn't have shiatsu?

Remember that shiatsu is principally used to enhance the healing process and create a state of well-being in the patient. There are a few circumstances where any interference, however subtle, may be unbeneficial. This is the case if you have a high fever, an infectious disease, cancer or some of the more serious heart conditions, while the effects of shiatsu will be limited if you are under strong drug medication or the influence of alcohol. However, shiatsu may be helpful in changing these more serious conditions if it is combined with dietary advice during a long course of treatment.

If surgery is necessary for certain conditions, shiatsu will be a helpful supplement in the recovery process. It is particularly advantageous in the case of hip replacements, broken bones, sports injuries and spinal problems, as well as surgery for digestive, reproductive and respiratory conditions. The time to be allowed before shiatsu can begin after surgery depends upon the seriousness of the operation; you should liaise with both your therapist and doctor in these circumstances.

Should I ask my doctor about receiving shiatsu?

These days an increasing number of doctors are aware of the limitations of allopathic medicine and are willing to refer patients to other therapists. There are, however, a large number of uninformed doctors around who have never heard of shiatsu, let alone know of its usefulness. It would therefore be most difficult for them to advise you on shiatsu; in such circumstances you would have to make your own decision.

Ideally, though, your doctor should always be consulted, as he or she may wish to notify the shiatsu therapist concerning your medical case history. If this is the case you will have to give your doctor permission to do so as your file is confidential. This is also the case in shiatsu; confidentiality is vitally important in establishing a trusting relationship between patient and therapist.

2
THE ENERGY SYSTEM

The word energy might make you think about fuel – fuel for your car, central heating, gas lighter or motor mower. The average person doesn't usually think of the oxygen we breathe or the food we eat as 'fuel' for our bodies. But every living organism needs this fuel to survive, and the quality and quantity of fuel influences our daily activity.

So, energy is fuel and fuel is energy. The two are inseparable. As referred to in Chapter 1, the energy of the body is distributed to all our cells, muscles, bones and organs through a system of electromagnetically charged channels called meridians. These meridians act like an irrigation system, allowing the free flow of energy to the crops or, in the case of animals such as ourselves, the organs. These meridians can be seen more tangibly in plant life than in animals. Look at a leaf for example; you will see vein-like lines branching out from the stem to the peripheries of the leaf. The energy flow comes from the centre and is distributed to the outside. These lines are the meridians of the leaf. The life-force of the plant travels through the energy system of the structure and 'pushes' fluids to the peripheries.

ZANG AND FU ORGANS

The human body is controlled by the vital organs and their energetic and physiological functions. The organs each have a different quality of energetic movement and responsibility. The balanced functioning of the body's metabolism depends on the compatibility of the organs as part of the whole body system and on their not being individual parts separate in their functions.

The organs do not simply consist of their physical structures; more importantly we should also take account of their responsibilities and their energetic functions. In the case of the liver, for example, not only does it have the physiological function of digesting fatty acid and helping elsewhere in digestion, but it has the energetic function of determining organisational skills, one's humour, level of patience, and other personality traits such as anger and frustration. Energetically, it nurtures the energy of the heart and small intestine and controls the balance of body vigour, sight and the function and general health of the muscles.

The Chinese did not think of the organs as being merely structures made up of condensed cells compacted into a recognisable shape; the function of each organ had a special relationship with the rest of the metabolism. Their concepts were not limited to what could be seen alone. In the case of the heart constrictor, for example, which is not a recognisable structure in the body, this energetic function controls the environment of the heart within its protective sac, the pericardium. It also relates to the emotions which affect the heart organ and acts as a protective 'buffer' for the heart against the flood of different emotional stresses that you may be subjected to daily.

In Oriental medicine the organs are categorised into two types; there are six *zang* organs and six *fu* organs. The *zang* organs are the harder, denser organs, namely the liver, heart, lungs, kidneys, spleen and heart constrictor; the *fu* organs are the softer more expanded organs, namely the gallbladder, small intestine, large intestine, bladder, stomach and triple heater. This last organ, like its pair, the heart constrictor, is not a structure and refers to certain functions of the energy; in particular it regulates the metabolism, the distribution of energy to the peripheries and controls the heating system of the body.

The energy required for the proper maintenance and functioning of these organs is distributed and regulated by the meridian system. There are 12 meridians, one for each organ function. These are, in order of the way the meridians connect with one another, the lung, large intestine, stomach, spleen/pancreas (this is considered the same organ function and is treated as one meridian), heart, small intestine, bladder, kidney, heart constrictor, triple heater, gallbladder and liver. The lung is considered to be the starting point for the meridian cycle of energy flow. This is because it is through the mouth and nose that we breathe in fresh energy, previously referred to as *ki*. This is the first stimulation response in birth. The baby exhales to release the last essence of the womb environment (internal existence) and takes in fresh *ki* from its new environment (outside existence); from this starting point, the baby has to depend on its own energetic function to maintain body balance. The energy circulates throughout the meridian system from the lung meridian to the liver, completing the cycle back to the lung. It is a complete circuit.

EXTRAORDINARY VESSELS

In order that natural adjustments to this basic system can occur when required, there are a further eight subsystems or extraordinary meridians known as vessels. As regards shiatsu, of the eight vessels the most important in their influence are the governing vessel and the conception vessel. These are responsible for the control and regulation of the energy circulating throughout the meridian system, and make necessary adjustments when excesses or deficiencies in the yin/yang balance of the body occur.

The energy flow is continuous and it is the quality and quantity of that energy which is changeable. Deficiencies and excesses in any part of the system determine your state of health. We are born with what is called original *ki*, which is stored in the kidneys; this is the energy we have acquired from our parents and is also thought of as the ancestral spirit of your family. It is this energy which is the most difficult to change, and it is thought that once the original *ki* is depleted, you die.

YIN AND YANG

If you live in accordance with the laws of nature and do not abuse yourself with all the extremes of modern living such as reliance on medicinal and illegal drugs, alcohol and processed foods, then the quality of your *ki* is maintained. Disregard your natural instincts for survival and degeneration begins.

The Chinese medical system follows a fundamental principle; that is, that everything is affected by and is part of a phenomena of nature known as yin and yang. These terms are used to describe the complementary yet opposing vibrational forces of nature which are responsible for the creation and continuance of everything in existence, including both animate and inanimate objects. This is the process of change and it must be realised that everything changes because energy by nature is ephemeral. Night turns to day and back to night again. The seasons move in a continuous cycle of change. All things in nature are born, live and then die, to nurture new life. Rocks are broken down by weather or tidal influences again to go through the process of conglomeration over millions of years. Trees grow, die and decay, to refertilise the soil for new growth. The examples are endless.

Have you ever thought why some vegetables grow above ground level and others below? The former are influenced by the predominance of yin, rising energy 'pushing' the main body of the vegetable such as a lettuce, for example, above ground level. The below-ground vegetables are influenced by the predominance of yang, descending energy 'pushing' the body deeper into the ground. Both natural forces always exist together and it is the varying degree of predominance which determines your health. Yin and yang are not good or bad; they merely show energy movement influenced in one way or another. If there is an imbalance in the yin and yang relationship within an organism then this disharmony is synonymous with a condition of dis-ease, a state where there is no

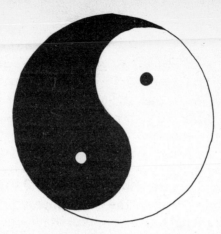

longer 'ease' or balance. The Taoist symbol above (the *tao* meaning The Way) is descriptive of this relationship.

Twelve principles of nature
- One Infinity manifests itself in complementary and antagonistic tendencies, yin and yang.
- Yin and yang are manifested continuously.
- Yin represents centrifugality, yang centripetality.
- Yin and yang together produce all phenomena.
- Yin attracts yang, yang attracts yin.
- Yin repels yin, yang repels yang.
- All phenomena are ephemeral.
- Nothing is solely yin or yang; everything is composed of both in varying degrees.
- Nothing is neuter; either yin or yang predominates.
- Large yin attracts small yin, large yang attracts small yang.
- Extreme yin produces yang; extreme yang produces yin.
- All manifestations are yang at the centre and yin at the surface.

THE MERIDIAN NATURES

The meridians are divided into categories of yin and yang. This means that a meridian described as yin is

Some features of yin and yang

Yin	Yang
Coldness	Hotness
Earth	Heaven
Female	Male
Expansion	Contraction
Centrifugal force	Centripetal force
Darkness	Light
Passive	Active
Surface	Deep
Exterior	Interior
Hollow	Solid
Front	Back
Ascending and vertical	Descending, horizontal
Longer	Shorter
Thinner	Thicker
Damp	Dry
Soft	Hard
Open	Closed
Separation	Gathering
More psychological	More physical
More spiritual	More social
Vegetable quality	Animal quality
Lighter	Heavier
Decomposition	Development
Sympathetic nervous system	Parasympathetic nervous system
Space	Time

predominantly influenced by this force and nurtures a yin function but has qualities of its opposite, yang. The meridians are paired, one being yin, the other yang. This reflects the true balance of nature, the dynamic complementary/antagonistic relationship of opposites. The yin meridians are located in the anterior and medial, more yin, soft side of the body, with the exception of the stomach meridian. The yang meridians are in the posterior and lateral, more yang, harder area. The yin meridian energy flows in an upward direction and the yang downward. The yin/yang balance of the meridian pairs are as follows:

• Lungs and large intestine

- Spleen/pancreas and stomach
- Heart and small intestine
- Bladder and kidney
- Heart constrictor and triple heater
- Liver and gall bladder

All of the meridians either start or end in the hands or feet and connect with the centre of the body. There are six pairs of meridians, three pairs in the arms and three pairs in the legs. The extraordinary vessels run through the centre of the body.

The Chinese thought of the meridians and their related organs in a conceptual sense, giving them official duties as in a government. When the various 'governmental departments' cooperate with one another there is harmony in the land. If one or several departments become disorganised or imbalanced then dissent and chaos result.

The book *The Yellow Emperor's Classic of Internal Medicine* is a partial translation of the ancient Chinese medical text the *Nei Ching*. It gives an enlightening description of the 'official duties'.

The Yellow Emperor said, 'I desire to hear how it is possible that the twelve viscera send each other that which is precious and that which is worthless.' Ch'i Po [the court physician], answered, 'How can I best answer this question? May I ask you to follow these words. The heart is like the minister of the monarch who excels through insight and understanding; the lungs are the symbol of the interpretation and conduct of the official jurisdiction and regulation; the liver has the function of a military leader who excels in his strategic planning; the gall bladder occupies the position of an important and upright official who excels through his decision and judgement; the middle of the thorax (the part between the breasts) is like the official of the centre who guides the subjects in their joys and pleasures; the stomach acts as the official of the public granaries and grants the five tastes; the lower intestines

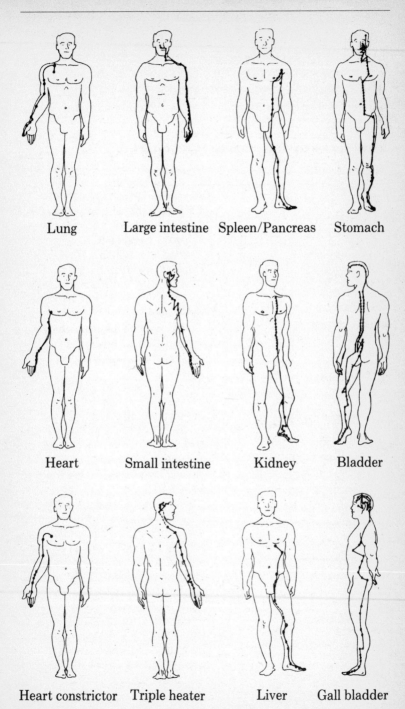

Lung   Large intestine   Spleen/Pancreas   Stomach

Heart   Small intestine   Kidney   Bladder

Heart constrictor   Triple heater   Liver   Gall bladder

are like the officials who propagate the Right Way of Living, and they generate evolution and change; the small intestines are like the officials who are trusted with riches, and they create changes of the physical substance; the kidneys are like the officials who do

Functions of the twelve meridians

Meridian	Function
Lungs	Interpretation and regulation. Exchanges material between outside and inside. Official in charge of jurisdiction.
Large intestine	Transmission. Official generating elimination and exchange.
Stomach	Assimilation. Controls the storage and digestion. Official in charge of the granary.
Spleen	Transformation and nourishment. Transportation of digestive enzymes. Official also in charge of storage.
Heart	Awareness and communication. Minister of the monarch; has insight and understanding.
Small intestine	Conversion. Official in charge of the treasury. Converts food into energy.
Bladder	Purification. Official in charge of storage of the overflow and fluid secretions.
Kidney	The water metabolism. Vitality and direction. Officials who do the energetic work.
Heart constrictor	Regulation and circulation of energy. Official of joy and pleasure.
Triple heater	Protection. Transportation and metabolic activity. Official who plans construction.
Gallbladder	Distribution and decision making. Official with good judgment and decisions.
Liver	Storage and organisation. Official in charge of planning.

energetic work, and they excel through their ability and cleverness; the burning spaces are like the officials who plan the construction of ditches and sluices, and they create waterways; the groins and bladder are like the magistrates of a region or district, they store the overflow and the fluid secretions which serve to regulate vaporisation. These twelve officials should not fail to assist one another.'

CONTROLLING FUNCTIONS OF THE ORGANS

There are a number of relationships between the energetic functions of organs and their physiological functions. The following refer to the *zang* organs, but can be considered to affect their respective paired organs.

- **Controls exerted on the viscera:**
  The heart controls the pulse.
  The lungs control the skin.
  The liver controls the muscles.
  The spleen controls the flesh (this includes the lips).
  The kidneys control the bones and nails.
- **External conditions affecting the viscera:**
  Heat injures the heart.
  Cold injures the lungs.
  Wind injures the liver.
  Humidity injures the spleen.
  Dryness injures the kidneys.
- **Spiritual resources controlled by the viscera:**
  The liver controls the soul.
  The heart controls the spirit.
  The spleen controls the ideas.
  The lungs control the inferior or animal spirit.
  The kidneys control the willpower.
- **The effects of flavours on the body:**
  Excess of salty flavour hardens the pulse.
  Excess of bitter flavour withers the skin.
  Excess of pungent flavour knots the muscles.
  Excess of sour flavour toughens the flesh.
  Excess of sweet flavour causes aches in the bones.

- **Fluid secretions connected with the viscera:**
  Sweat connected with the heart.
  Mucus connected with the lungs.
  Tears connected with the liver.
  Saliva connected with the spleen.
  Urine connected with the kidneys.

PRESSURE POINTS - WHAT DO THEY DO?

The Japanese word used to describe a pressure point is
tsubo. The literal English translation means vase, a
container for water, which is synonymous with energy in
shiatsu. Referring back to Chapter 1 and the description
of the meridian channels as an irrigation system, the *tsubo*
are like inspection points on the irrigation pipelines. From
these points the state of flow of the energy in a particular
meridian can be determined. Each meridian has a varying
number of *tsubo* and there are in excess of 700 *tsubo* in the
human body. Each *tsubo* reflects the state of health and
energy quality of its related organ. Pain is the most
common indicator of energy distortion.

The *tsubo* are points of tangible electrical charge, and
messages passed through the meridian system create
subtle changes in the intensity of the electrical charge at
any given *tsubo* location. These points can be used for
both diagnosis and treatment, as they are a reflection of
the internal functioning of the body systems. Thousands
of years of Oriental medical practice have shown the
effectiveness of this form of treatment for releasing
blocked energy, thereby relieving the patient of previously
persisting symptoms. The Oriental mind is such that the
usage of acupuncture and shiatsu is naturally accepted as
valid therapy, on the simple basis that they work. On the
other hand, the strenuously logical Western mind cannot
grasp the concept of something working unless the reasons
for its working are clear.

The *tsubo* may be seen to have a nerve reflex action
which displays an external reaction to an internal
malfunctioning. This is found usually as pain, stiffness,

numbness, fatty deposits, discolouration, cold or hot
areas, skin eruptions or rashes, moles, freckles or
pigmentation along any given meridian pathway.
Indications such as pimples, rashes and warts show a
more acute condition reflex, whereas moles and freckles N
are a reflection of past functional traumas such as high
fever in childhood. The *tsubo* is part of the communication
system between the principle energy of the meridian
which feeds and nurtures the organs, bones, flesh,
muscles, subcutaneous and connective tissue and the
skin, as well as all the cells of the body.

The therapist will determine whether to treat the *tsubo*
in the immediate area of a symptom or to go further away
from this location to another reflex area which has been
affected and will in turn affect the symptoms. The *tsubo*
in the area of a chronic elbow problem, for example, need
to be treated, but may not require as much emphasis as
the *tsubo* in the legs relating to the liver and gallbladder
energy which controls the muscles and joints generally. It
is not satisfactory to look only at the symptom location:
the causation must be determined and treated to change a
symptom permanently. Pressure applied to the *tsubo* will
create the movement of electrical messages throughout
the meridian and nervous system to be received by the
brain for interpretation. A response will then be felt back
at the *tsubo*. To press any *tsubo* will transmit a subtle
energy movement throughout all 12 meridians and vessels.
This reaction is likened to throwing a stone into a pool of
water; from the point of contact the vibration (ripples)
move to the periphery of the pond and return to the
original contact point. (The effect of the nervous system is
discussed in Chapter 3.) When the *tsubo* is accurately
diagnosed and treated, the original symptom of pain or
stiffness will disappear, showing that the energy blockages
have been released and the natural healing process of the
body is activated.

SYMPTOMS AND THE MERIDIANS

Symptoms are merely a manifestation of energy movement. The frequency and seriousness of the symptoms changes from person to person, depending upon their individual fitness level. The body reacts in many different ways. Your age, stress level, physical and mental fitness will create variations from one person to another. Basically, the less fit you are the more symptoms you are likely to have. Everyone has symptoms of one sort or another, which may be on a physical, emotional or psychological level.

Most people subconsciously seem to enjoy having symptoms. What would your reaction be if you said to someone 'How are you today?' and they replied 'I feel perfect'? End of conversation, that's for sure. There is no invitation given for you to enquire about this person's symptoms. It is usually more interesting to know what someone's problems are than why they feel so great. Sad, but true.

Your symptom may be a sore toe, backache, migraine, depression or confusion. The actual symptom itself is not paramount; it may be any factor which draws your attention and distracts your normal activity. These energy changes are part of the continual cycle of life and so we shouldn't be surprised to realise that as soon as one symptom disappears, another conveniently replaces it. The symptoms are the end result of some 'action' elsewhere in the body. Surface signs such as rashes and fatty deposits are a reflection of internal disorders. In shiatsu we look for the cause of a symptom or set of symptoms, for the 'action' which has stimulated the symptomatic 'reaction' to appear. Finding the cause is the true essence of proper diagnosis and treatment, leading to the successful elimination of the problem.

The cause is reflected in the meridian/organ function. These same functions may be related to a variety of symptoms as an indicator of energy distortion. Skin eruptions, for example, are associated primarily with lung

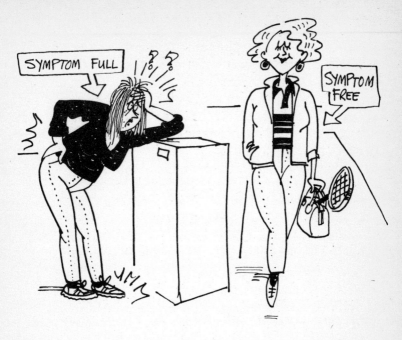

energy dysfunction, as is certainly the case in asthma syndrome eczema. This is a clear example of the 'outside' being a mirror of the condition of the 'inside'. Instead of merely applying external remedies, treatment of the lung meridian and other affected meridians and areas will speed the recovery process and the skin condition will change accordingly.

Because there are always several contributing factors involved in the appearance of any symptom, there will be more than just one organ function involved. Think of the body as a set of dominoes; should one domino be disturbed and fall, all the other dominoes will also react. All parts of the body must be functioning and co-existing in harmony for the 'whole' to be happy. You may, for instance, have a frozen shoulder but find that your therapist seemingly gives a small amount of attention to this area, concentrating instead on your legs and abdomen. In fact your frozen shoulder will probably be the result of liver or heart disturbances, which need rectification.

The therapist continually looks for areas where there is an excess of energy: that is, where the energy has condensed or gathered, coming from elsewhere in the body. This energy may become stuck and immobilise the area. The other condition looked for is that of deficiency: that is, areas where the energy is lacking and has dispersed to other parts of the body. Here the area lacks vitality or lifeforce. It is the subsequent energy rebalancing of these areas of excess and deficiency which makes shiatsu so effective. Because it is the energy which has created the physical structure, the energy must in turn be rebalanced to change any distortions in the structure. For example, mechanical adjustments to joints will immediately change the structural imbalance; however, unless the supporting energy is also rebalanced, the structure will again distort and the symptoms recur. Correct the causative imbalance in the energy system and the structural system will change, more slowly, but permanently.

SOME COMMON SYMPTOM/ENERGY RELATIONSHIPS

Lungs
- **Psychological** – depression, over anxiety, difficulty in relationships, hypersensitivity, stubbornness, mental inflexibility, inability to 'let go' of emotional disturbance.
- **Physical** – distension and or tightness of the chest, coughing and fatigue, susceptibility to colds and flu, asthma, bronchitis, abnormal body temperature changes, tendency to faint, shoulder and upper back pains, pains or stiffness in the elbow and palm side of the forearm, sunken or hollow cheeks, sagging or dry skin, skin eruptions, stiff or weak thumb.

Large intestine
- **Psychological** – insular, mental inflexibility, lacking determination, dominating others, general

dissatisfaction, always disappointed, over dependency on others, physical depression, sloppiness, holding grudges.
- **Physical** – nasal congestion, frontal headaches, excessive ear wax, overeating, poor sleeping, snoring, constipation or diarrhoea, throat pain, upper arm pain, stiffness in the shoulder and upper chest, sensitivity to temperature, sagging skin, pale facial colour, swollen lower lip, yellowing of eyeballs, flaccid buttocks.

Stomach
- **Psychological** – blameful of others, cynical and suspicious, thinking too much, worrying excessively, moody, reluctance to adapt to changes.
- **Physical** – gastric problems, overeating, nervous and restless, coldness in front of body and stomach organ, menstrual irregularities, poor appetite, anaemic, dry skin, tendency to high fever and sweating, upper lip rash and swelling, knee pains, tightness in the solar plexus, irregular eating times.

Spleen
- **Psychological** – self pity, cold personal relationships, restless, over anxious, timid, not sharing worries, usually alone, critical, general dissatisfaction, poor memory, hesitant, meticulous concern for detail.
- **Physical** – nausea and vomiting, tight root of tongue, thirsty, anaemia, irregular gastric acid production, irregular appetite, stomach inflammations, whole body tired and stiff, swelling in hips, knees or inside thighs, menstrual difficulties, sensitive and stiff navel, puffiness or darkish colouring of temples, rough skin, heel inflammation or cracking.

Heart
- **Psychological** – susceptible to stress and nervous tension, mental fatigue, communication difficulties, nervous laughter, over excitable, hypertense, erratic

changes of mind and mood, restless, lacking willpower, suppressing emotions.
- **Physical** – angina, chest constriction, stiffness in upper arms, yellowish eyeballs, sweaty palms, poor appetite, tight solar plexus, palpitations, hysteria, left shoulder pain, pain between shoulder blades, root of tongue feeling tight, increased or decreased sensitivity to temperature changes, poor circulation, red facial colour, swollen purplish nose.

Small intestine
- **Psychological** – introverted, thinking too much, suppresses sorrow, oversensitive, great patience, strongly affected by shock and anger, over concentration on detail, difficulty on concentrating on more than one thing at a time, changeable mind, overworks.
- **Physical** – poor digestion, poor circulation in extremities, pain or swelling in cheeks, scapular pain, loose flesh, poor muscle tone, erratic assimilation of nutrition, sciatic and lumbar pains, bloated abdomen, menstrual cycle irregularities, cervical vertebrae stiffness and restricted rotation, swollen or discoloured middle lower lip.

Bladder
- **Psychological** – easily frightened, paranoia, takes no risks, insecure, poor concentration, anxiety and restlessness, complaining, neurotic, over concentration and concern for small detail.
- **Physical** – low back and sacral palms, swelling or stiffness, dysfunction of autonomic nervous system, poor concentration, nosebleeds, stiff neck, posterior headaches, sluggish circulation in legs and abdomen, stiffness in back of knees, prostate or bladder and womb inflammations, cystitis, epilepsy, excessive tearing, pain from fifth toe to heel.

Kidney

- **Psychological** – fearful, defensive, timid, insecure, frustrated, violence coming from fear, pessimistic, lacking determination, hesitating, no willpower, constant complaining, can't complete things.
- **Physical** – loss of appetite, erratic or low libido, abnormally darkish facial colour, puffiness or darkness under the eyes, ringing in the ears, dry tongue, throat inflammation and dryness, chronic diarrhoea, blood in sputum or urine, reproductive organ problems, lacking general vitality.

Heart constrictor

- **Psychological** – self-protective nature, fear of heights, easy tearfulness, reluctant to express oneself, absent-minded, nervous in groups, hypersensitive.
- **Physical** – pain in front of heart, cramping in forearm and elbow, restless sleep, tonsillitis, low or high blood pressure, tingling sensation in fingers, cardiac dysfunctions, poor circulation to extremities, colitis, palpitations, dizziness, stiffness in solar plexus.

Triple Heater

- **Psychological** – disorganised thinking due to fatigue, obsessive, over cautious, tense, anxious, excessive worrying, need to get things his or her own way, spoiled, hypersensitive.
- **Physical** – cheek and posterior ear pains, shoulder and upper arm joint pains, deafness, swollen larynx, poor lymphatic drainage, sensitivity to changes in humidity and temperature, regularly catches cold, prone to inflammation, excessive sweating, abnormal blood pressure, pressure behind eyes, inflammation in womb, poor circulation in lower limbs.

Gallbladder

- **Psychological** – indecisive, impatient, taking on too many responsibilities, overly excitable, lacking determination, always hurrying, excessive

concentration, low motivation, fatigued after
emotional outbursts, mental fatigue.
- **Physical** – fatigue, poor digestion, stiff joints, swollen
lymph nodes in neck and armpit, recurring chills and
fevers, migraine headaches at side of head or behind
eyes, bitter taste in mouth, swelling above shoulder
blades, tired eyes, gallstones, dizziness, mucus
discharge in eyes, poor sleep, small appetite but
unable to lose weight.

Liver
- **Psychological** – argumentative, abusive, revengeful,
complaining, impatient, suppressed anger at world,
little humour, loud nature, lacking determination,
prone to violent outbursts, generally bored, needing
constant excitement through change.
- **Physical** – overeating, weakness in joints, nausea
and vomiting due to indigestion, distension of middle
organ area, accumulated fatigue due to excess vitality
for work, prostate problems, poor muscle flexibility,
puffy or discoloured in area between the eyebrows,
frontal headache, tightness in movement, liver
malfunctioning, lumbar and middle back pain,
impotence or lack of sexual energy, cannot maintain
an erection, female reproductive organ inflammation.

Conception vessel
- **Psychological** – difficulty in sexual relationships,
low self-esteem, overly self-protective, difficulty
communicating with others.
- **Physical** – diseases of genito-urinary system, hernia,
coldness in abdomen, bloating of abdomen,
bedwetting, impotence, menstrual disorders, stomach
pains, gastrointestinal disorders, bladder infections,
heart related problems, spiritual unrest.

Governing vessel
- **Psychological** – nervous emotional state,
hypersensitive, rigidity in thinking, own opinion is best.

- **Physical** – pains along spinal column, headaches, back pains, diseases of central nervous system, mentally disturbed, intestinal bleeding, haemorrhoids, anorexia, epilepsy, multiple sclerosis, paralytic diseases.

3
SHIATSU AND THE NERVOUS SYSTEM

The 'nervous system response', as it relates to shiatsu, was an explanation first used by a well-known shiatsu teacher, Saul Goodman. It is sometimes difficult to explain to a layperson about the actual mechanics of shiatsu and this approach provides some clarity. The Western mind needs to see things in a logical and analytical form, which is why it often has difficulties understanding Oriental medicine. Eastern medicine seldom emphasises a logical basis for interpretation, and

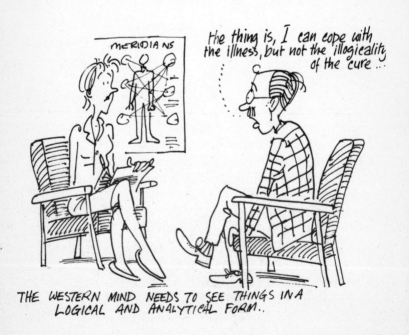

THE WESTERN MIND NEEDS TO SEE THINGS IN A LOGICAL AND ANALYTICAL FORM..

is usually based on thousands of years of clinical research experience and not the accepted Western approach of scientific testing. This of course does not make it any better or worse than Western medicine, only less logical, to Westerners.

THE CENTRAL AND AUTONOMIC NERVOUS SYSTEMS

Let us proceed from the physiological point of view. The nervous system is divided into two main systems, the central nervous system (CNS) and the autonomic nervous system (ANS). The CNS is in charge of our more 'conscious' activity; it is the CNS which is now controlling your hand movements as you hold and turn the pages of this book – your hand and eye coordination at work. This system can be improved and maintained with both physical and mental exercise. The CNS is our intellectually developed decision-maker, our modern-day caretaker of the body's conscious functions. The major components of the CNS are the brain and the spinal cord, with nerves attached. Messages in the form of electrical impulses pass along the nerve fibres to and from the brain. This system functions largely as a result of reflex, sensation and conscious decision.

The ANS is our 'unconscious' control and relates to both physical and emotional functions. This is our primal instinct in operation. It is subdivided into the sympathetic and parasympathetic systems. The ANS regulates the organs of blood circulation, respiration, digestion, excretion and reproduction, controlling the functions and organs over which we have no voluntary control. For example, the movement of food through the digestive tract is called peristalsis, and consists of complementary actions of expansion and contraction to create movement of food particles in a squeezing wave-like movement. It is wholly reflex, independent of the brain function. It is interesting to note that peristalsis is often stimulated into action during a shiatsu treatment.

THE ALPHA STATE

The nerves of the sympathetic section of the autonomic nervous system have the effect of increasing body activity, while the parasympathetic nerves slow down the body activity. In shiatsu we wish to induce a state of relaxation in the patient. Therefore the body functions need to slow down and become calm. The parasympathetic response is to allow the patient to relax, become open and non-resisting to the changes that are occurring. This enables a simple unification of the mind and body. At this point the patient goes into a semi-hypnotic state called the alpha state. We all go through this experience twice every day. It is the relaxed transition phase between when you lay down to go to sleep and the point at which you actually fall asleep. You are semi-conscious and aware of your surroundings but merely observing and not participating consciously in those surroundings. If a door closes you hear this but register it as not being a danger and drift off again. The same experience occurs as you go from deep sleep to full alertness in the morning. It is generally considered that sleeping tablets have the effect of bypassing this transition period, which is vitally important for restful sleep. And as many a sleeping pill user has found to their detriment, the more you use such pills, the more you need them.

QUESTIONS AND ANSWERS

Can I control my autonomic nervous system?
The person with a parasympathetic predominance in daily life is generally more calm and relaxed. This may be positive or negative, depending on your needs. Sometimes we need controlled tension to work effectively, and being too 'laid back' may be unsatisfactory. However, it is useful to be able to stimulate this predominance when necessary. Deep breathing is the simplest method of doing so. Deep breathing allows a greater quantity of oxygen to enter the bloodstream and creates a more alkaline, less acid

condition. When you feel tense and the body activity is increased by sympathetic system predominance, your heart races, your breathing is shallow and rapid, the abdomen tightens and your reactions are impaired. This is the prime environment in which ulcers can develop and is the time to breathe deeply and relax.

Can I feel my nervous system response during a shiatsu treatment?

In your shiatsu treatment you will initially feel the point where the therapist's thumb is applied. Your ANS will automatically determine whether this pressure is something to be fearful of and thus resist, or whether this touch is nurturing and 'needed'. The sympathetic system would defend the body against pain by creating a resistance, tensing the muscles as protection. Obviously, this won't be very relaxing, but in the hands of an experienced therapist even painful areas can be held and nurtured as energy is released. Some pain can be tolerated and can even be soothing, such as when you press your temples to relieve a headache. It hurts, but it is relieving; your body actually 'wants' this pain.

When you 'let go' during a treatment your parasympathetic system opens up and any emotional and

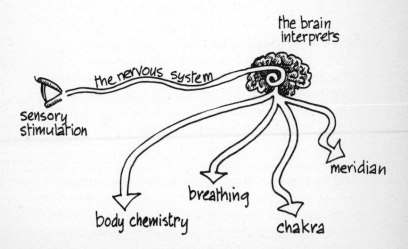

physical barriers melt away. If the therapist is applying pressure at two points, on the arm for example, you will no longer be able to feel the two separate areas of attention; your mind will drift and the two points become indistinguishable. This is what is called the 'switch', the point at which the sympathetic resistance is diminished and the ANS switches to parasympathetic predominance.

How does this relate to meridians?

As explained in Chapter 2, the meridians form the body's energy system and these electromagnetic pathways of energy connect the vital organs in a complete cycle of energy flow, the meridian cycle. By applying touch and penetrating pressure to the skin surface, the meridians can be tapped into, diagnosed and treated. The therapist will switch concentration from the physical anatomy to the energetic anatomy. Treating a point or area on the lung meridian, for example, will not only send a message to the brain via the nervous system: it will also create a movement or vibration in the energy field of the patient. As in the case of throwing a pebble into a pool of water, the vibrations move from the point of pressure to the periphery and then return, and it is this returning reaction which the therapist will 'listen' to, to determine whether the point or area has a deficiency or excess of energy. If the reaction is fast then there is an 'excess', if it is very slow then there is a 'deficiency'. The terms used to describe these conditions respectively are *jitsu* and *kyo*.

As the energy has created the structure, the energy is always considered to come before the structure. However, *ki* is also refreshed and produced by the vital organs, so if a particular organ is weakened then the energy it produces will be affected. This is the cycle of energy movement. The *ki* draws the blood to any given area of the body; by stimulating the meridians, as explained in Chapter 2, you can improve the energy flow and consequently the blood circulation will also improve. So, when we talk about stimulating the autonomic nervous system, it cannot really be separated from the energetic movement in the body; after all, the energy of the bladder meridian has created and now controls the nervous system function.

What is the aura?

The meridians are the pathways of energy, but are not the only means of energy function and movement. The whole body, the total organism, is made up of energy.

We have a physical border or barrier, the skin. This contains and limits the more dense physical body, but still allows the less tangible *ki* to move through the physical as well as the etheric sphere, the latter being the energy 'attached' to the body as a surrounding protective layer. This is sometimes referred to as the aura.

Most of us feel the presence of someone approaching as they are about to touch us. This reaction depends on your own self-awareness; and martial artists, for example, train themselves to react when another person's aura enters their own auric space. Have you ever been in a crowded room with your back to the door, and for no apparent reason you turn to face the door as a friend arrives? You simply 'feel' their presence. This auric energy force field can be photographed in a process called Kirlian photography.

Is energy only in the meridians?

Inside the body there is energy in all our living cells. When your therapist talks about heart energy, for example, he or she is not simply referring to the heart organ but to the energy affecting every blood vessel in your body. *Ki* is the basis of each cell, which is the physical structure talked about previously.

The membranes or fascia which surround the organs and nerves are packed with *ki*, acting as a protective layer for that organ. Whenever there is a distortion in the energy, there will subsequently appear a dysfunction in the organs, muscles and connective tissue in the area controlled by that *ki*. Messages of pain pass through the energy stored in the fascia to the nerves and then to the spinal cord. From here the message goes to the brain for interpretation. If there is a deficiency of energy in the fascia surrounding an organ, that organ may be easily damaged, for example by a heavy blow.

Is there a scientific explanation?

Because many forms of Oriental medicine are now widely used in the West there is more pressure being exerted by the medical profession for production of a scientific rationale as to how therapies such as acupuncture, shiatsu and reflexology actually work. It is the unfortunate difference between the Eastern and Western mind that Western logic cannot conceive that something can work unless it is known specifically why and how it does. The students of Oriental medicine such as myself take a different approach in interpreting Oriental medical theory and practice, keeping what is called a beginner's mind. A Zen master once stated, 'In the beginner's mind there are many possibilities, but in the expert's there are few.' Our expert Western minds do not really wish to accept that something works simply because it does work.

There has been a large amount of research into acupuncture which also applies to shiatsu. For example, the Peking Medical College did a great deal of work on pain control through *tsubo* stimulation, with very positive results. Of course, acupuncture as an anaesthetic is still used widely in both China and Japan during both major and minor surgery. To explain this there is the endorphin theory, which concludes that, by stimulating the *tsubo*, substances called endorphins are activated which suppress the pain signals normally transmitted to the brain through the central nervous system. Certainly in shiatsu this principle can be used directly to change the pain threshold, and is particularly useful in cases of sports or other traumatic injury; for example, the May 1988 edition of the *Midwives Chronicle* gave details of research into acupuncture and shiatsu and its effectiveness for pain relief during pregnancy and childbirth.

Whether there will ever be a satisfactory explanation of

shiatsu from a Western point of view is questionable. For the moment we have to accept the fact that it works, without a specific scientific explanation as to why.

Do we really need an explanation?

4
DIAGNOSIS – ART OR SCIENCE?

There is a simple and basic principle to follow in Oriental medical diagnosis; that is, everything changes, nothing is static. There is no escaping this natural process. We are all born, we live and we die.

It is this principle of observing natural changes that makes Oriental diagnosis more of an art than a science to the Western mind. In shiatsu, the therapist observes the energy of the patient for imbalances which may manifest as physical, emotional or psychological symptoms. This is the study of life phenomena.

The *Concise Oxford Dictionary* gives various meanings for the word 'science'. One such meaning relating to natural and physical science is 'knowledge dealing with material phenomena and based mainly on observation, experimentation and induction'. Oriental medicine, developed over thousands of years of case history, observation and clinical treatment, is a science in a different sense of the word.

It is the mental attitude or approach of the shiatsu therapist which differs greatly to that of the average allopathic doctor. The therapist learns to develop what is called *shoshin* in Japanese. This means beginner's mind, an attitude of observation and receptiveness. This attitude avoids the over intellectualising and judgmental attitudes that occur when strictly systematised logical thought is involved. When you consider yourself an expert in any field you may close yourself off to new ideas because these may be contradictory to your own. This can create dangerous situations. With the beginner's mind you are eager to learn, in this case all about your patient, and remain open to accept information which may appear contradictory. The same symptoms which are seen in a number of people may each have a totally different cause and require a substantially altered clinical approach to that of the others.

Shiatsu diagnosis is thus more of an art than what is usually considered to be science. Just as an artist will sit and observe a landscape, absorbing the essence of its qualities before beginning to sketch, the shiatsu therapist will observe the patient. The art here is to observe without 'looking'. By observing, we make ourselves open to information rather than strenuously looking for it and getting caught up in small details which may distract us from seeing the whole person and their strengths and weaknesses.

We've probably all been in the situation where we've lost something which we search for without success, then only find it when we stop looking for it. This is one of life's lessons.

TYPES OF DIAGNOSIS

Symptoms, posture, body language, emotions, reactions, verbal replies to questions, all may be perceived as part of the jigsaw puzzle of your life history. Gradually, as more and more information is received, the picture becomes clearer. Shiatsu diagnosis is not based on any one symptom or feature manifested by the patient, it is an accumulation of information which gives a composite impression of the patient's condition. Four types of diagnosis are used.

- *Bo-shin*, visual diagnosis.
- *Setsu-shin*, touch diagnosis.
- *Mon-shin*, question diagnosis.
- *Bun-shin*, senses diagnosis, including the use of intuition.

Visual diagnosis, *bo-shin.*
We all use this type of diagnosis unwittingly every day.

You might find yourself watching someone on the bus, in the street or at a party; you make a character diagnosis, and think 'I'd like to talk to that person.' Or maybe you'd think 'I'd hate to be trapped in a faulty elevator with him.' And have you ever noticed how some people look very pale or puffy in the face? Maybe they have bags under the eyes, and you assume they need some rest. The experienced observer can use these observations to formulate a diagnosis of a person's condition of health.

Similarly, your therapist will be observing you from the moment you walk in. How you walk, sit down, hold your head, cross your legs, maintain your posture, all supply information about your energetic balance or imbalances. Often the body language gives a clearer picture than the words you are saying. Picture someone sitting talking to you and saying what a relaxed open person they are; however their legs and arms are tightly crossed, their fists clenched and their jaw tight. Which impression of them would you be left with, that of a calm down-to-earth type, or a nervous, insecure type?

There are many areas of the body to look at – the face, posture, hands, feet, head and body hair, skin texture, muscle tone. The microcosm is a reflection of the macrocosm, the small view reflects the larger view. Look at the face, for example; have you ever wondered about those puffy bags under your eyes which get worse when you party or work too much and don't get enough sleep? Those bags are a reflection of the disrupted kidney energy and functions telling you to slow down. The face is like a map of the internal functions; the outside reflects the inside.

How does it work? The science of the hologram makes a useful analogy. A picture of an object is taken by a laser and this information is stored in a sheet of glass. The glass containing the three dimensional image can be broken and a tiny portion may be used to reconstitute the whole image again. The total information of the macrocosm is stored in the microcosm, as in the case of the face storing information about the whole body.

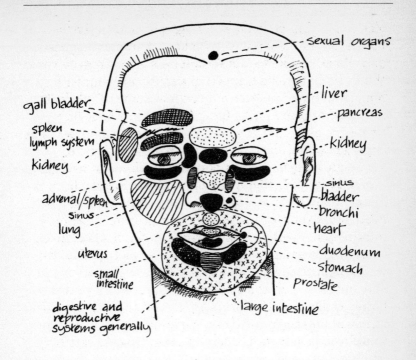

The diagram shows a face with areas labelled for different organs:

- sexual organs
- liver
- pancreas
- kidney
- sinus
- bladder
- bronchi
- heart
- duodenum
- stomach
- prostate
- large intestine
- gall bladder
- spleen lymph system
- kidney
- adrenal/spleen
- sinus
- lung
- uterus
- small intestine
- digestive and reproductive systems generally

Question diagnosis, *mon-shin*

Question diagnosis is obviously important. You will be asked questions by your therapist about your current health and the history of your health problems. It's very rare to find someone who just tells you of all the good periods of their life – 'Yes, well I was very healthy in 1986 and 1987. They were particularly good years.' The case history is usually full of all the bad times filled with pain and frustration.

But your symptoms are only part of the story requiring research. If you are seeking advice about your gallstones and it transpires that you have a high fatty acid intake in your diet, then your diet will also need some attention and gradual adjustment to rectify the situation. If you deal with the symptoms alone and ignore the underlying causatory factors, then you run the risk of the same, and usually worsened, symptoms arising again in the future. For example, if you get a migraine headache and it is always initiated by eating chocolate, (which admittedly will only be part of the cause), then it is obvious that chocolate should be dropped from your diet. If you persistently strain your back from incorrectly lifting objects, then you need to strengthen the back and retrain yourself to lift correctly.

Questions about past surgery, injuries or serious illnesses are important factors and may influence the treatment given. Some past illnesses can give an indication of the possible contributing factors in relation to your current condition. For example, a whiplash which occurred 10 or 15 years ago may only now create a painful and persistent symptom.

But it must always be remembered that we are very complex creatures and there need be no logical explanation for such events occurring.

Touch diagnosis, *setsu-shin*

Touch is the most positive and informative diagnostic tool in shiatsu. Your muscle tone, skin condition, lumps, moles, hairy patches, flexibility and pain response tell much about your health condition. If you lead a sedentary life, doing very little physical work or exercise, eating poor quality foods, and probably eating too much of them, then it is likely that you will carry excess weight. This excess weight will strain your skeletal system; it is designed for a certain natural body weight and more than this creates problems. If you have chronic back and neckache, have a serious look at your weight and general state of health.

Is your muscle tone far removed from what it was when you were younger? Certainly as we age our skin condition changes, but most of us age ourselves prematurely because of our lifestyles. One of the effects of shiatsu will be to improve your circulation and the secretion of the body's natural lubricating oils responsible for maintaining healthy skin and muscle tone. When the digestive function improves, so will your skin condition. Because of these changes, many patients look younger after a series of treatments, and may well have lost many stress-related lines in the face.

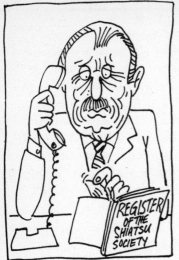 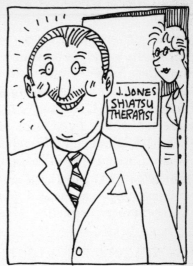

...MANY PATIENTS LOOK YOUNGER AFTER A SERIES OF TREATMENTS...

Senses diagnosis, *Bun-shin*

Often it is the senses, such as smell, hearing and intuition, which draw the therapist's attention to some possible imbalance. For example, a weakness in the lungs may create a rasping or wheezing sound in the voice. Stagnation in the bowel usually produces a pungent and sometimes putrefying smell on the breath.

The voice tells the therapist about other conditions. There are five common types of voice, each relating to different conditions.

- Nervous laughter shows an imbalance in fire energy (heart and small intestine functions).
- A sing-song voice relates to the soil energy (stomach, spleen/pancreas functions).
- A whining or weepish voice relates to the metal energy (lungs and large intestine functions).
- A groaning or gargling voice relates to the water energy (kidney and bladder functions).
- And a shouting or sharp voice relates to the wood energy (liver and gallbladder functions).

(See Chapter 5 for more details about the elemental energies.)

Still under this category of diagnosis comes the least scientific, but often most important, diagnostic tool, intuition. Your therapist will rely heavily upon his or her experience and developed 'gut' feeling about your condition and its causes. The intuitive decision simply directs the therapist to look into a certain aspect of your physical, emotional or psychological health. This is really where the concept of the beginner's mind is paramount. Being open to insights without logical analytical deduction requires practice. Trusting your intuition requires that you believe in yourself.

WHICH IS BETTER, ORIENTAL OR ALLOPATHIC DIAGNOSIS?

Often these days patients are informed by their doctors that there is nothing that can be done for their chronic neckache, their menstrual problem, their migraine, backache or some other undiagnosable symptom. What happens now? Live with the pain and frustration or seek a second opinion? Most people, in fact, seek several opinions and then approach a shiatsu or other natural health therapist. It is at this time that the oriental theory of diagnosis gives a greater insight into the cause and therefore treatment of the symptoms.

Probably 80 per cent of patients I see for back disorders have been through the whole allopathic system and been told there is nothing physically wrong. There obviously is something amiss, but they don't know the cause unless physical damage can be found. It is at this stage we enter the wider category of stress-related symptoms. I once had a patient whose chronic low backache flared up every time she argued with her husband. By giving her shiatsu to help her deal with her stress, and giving dietary and exercise advice, her back improved and so did her relationship.

The amount of time your GP can spend with you differs

greatly from that given by the shiatsu therapist. Have you ever been with your GP for longer than 10 minutes? Even that is a longer session than most. In contrast, your shiatsu session is usually an hour or more. It is not a question of incompetence, just the time made available. The other main advantage of a shiatsu diagnosis is that the emotional and psychological state, and not just the physical, is always taken into consideration in treatment. A prognosis of your future health is also more obvious because the energy system is seen as the primary focus; the prognosis is not discoloured by the appearance or absence of symptoms.

However, your shiatsu therapist will probably suggest you see your own doctor if he or she finds a problem which needs allopathic medical attention. For instance, if I suspect there may be a tumour or a cyst in the organs of a woman's reproductive system, then I will suggest they have a gynaecological examination.

DIAGNOSIS OF BODY AREAS

The head, face and neck

As seen in the diagram on page 49, different facial areas indicate a variety of organ functions or dysfunctions. Those sunken grey coloured cheeks seen on some people are an indication of lung disorders; such people will probably also have a more sunken upper chest, and shoulders coming forward as the chest collapses. Red cheeks may indicate an excess of energy in the lungs and general tightness in the chest. The red facial colour is also an indication of circulation and possible heart disorders.

The shape of the head itself gives an indication as to whether the person is of a more practical or intellectual type. The square-shaped head usually goes with the practical personality of someone who works with their hands in some manner, the longer or more vertical head type indicating a more intellectualising or spiritual character who works more by thinking and analysing matters than manual work. If a person sits or walks with the head always leaning forward, then their centre of gravity is too high because too much attention goes into thinking; they are likely to suffer neck, head and back pain from stress.

The neck itself is part of our communication mechanism as it contains the throat energy centre responsible for speech. Tightness often occurs in the throat when you feel nervous or tense about a situation. Pain or tension in the back of the neck is an indication of bladder energy problems. The cervical vertebrae of the neck are closely related in design and function to the lumbar or low back vertebrae. In the majority of cases a stiff neck will be accompanied by a stiff or painful lower back. The outer posterior neck, to the side of the neck, reflects more the function of the gallbladder and small intestine meridians. For example, if you were in a car accident and you were hit from the side then the neck whiplash you are likely to sustain will cause problems in the gallbladder meridian located in this area. The neck also becomes stressed when you hold in anger or tension.

Arms, shoulders and hands
The tops of the shoulders and the position of the shoulders provide information about the digestive and respiratory functions. Pimples on the shoulder are generally a sign of attempted elimination of toxins by the digestive system, and also usually indicate overeating. The right shoulder is related to the function of the liver, while the left is related to the functions of the heart and spleen. Many people have a bilateral imbalance, with one shoulder higher or lower than the other.

The elbows indicate middle organ function, the right referring to the gallbladder and liver primarily and the left to the spleen and stomach functions. This is helpful in determining the causative factors in 'tennis elbow', for example.

The forearms generally show the conditions of the lungs and breasts as well as the intestines. Puffiness, discolouration along a meridian pathway, cysts or fatty nodules indicate problems in these areas. A common example is seen in women with a fatty deposit in the middle inside forearm, as there are often associated breast lumps. The wrists reflect the state of the reproductive organ function; swelling or pain in the wrists, together with abnormal discolouration, are all signs of imbalances.

The hands and fingers often retain stress. Purpling or redness in the extremities – both fingers and toes – are an indication of the overconsumption of yin type foods such as sugar, alcohol, chemicalised foods and caffeine. Discolouration or puffiness around the root of the thumb indicate intestinal problems, the right side reflecting the state of the ascending colon and the left the descending colon. The arm meridians of heart, small intestine, triple heater, heart constrictor, large intestine and lung either begin or end in the fingers; if you have stiffness, pain, discolouration or any other abnormality in a finger, it can be related to the particular meridian function. Work on the meridian will help adjust the problem. The fingernails are controlled by the energy of the kidneys, which also control the bone quality.

The torso and abdomen

The chest and upper back reflect the energy of the heart and lungs as well as the patient's ability to deal with emotions – this is the heart centre, the seat of our communication with others and of our social activity. Have you ever been told to get a problem off your chest?

The biceps or frontal area of the upper arms also reflects the lung condition, while the rear or triceps area of the upper arm indicates the heart function. Many people who generally overeat and lack regular exercise have puffiness and fat accumulation in this area – a sign of over-nourishment.

The abdomen, or *hara* as it is called in Japanese, is a diagnostic map in itself. It gives the practitioner an indication of the imbalances in the meridians. The quality of the energy of all 12 meridians can be felt in this area.

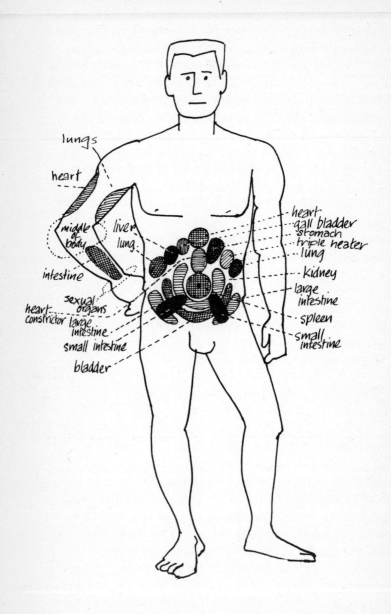

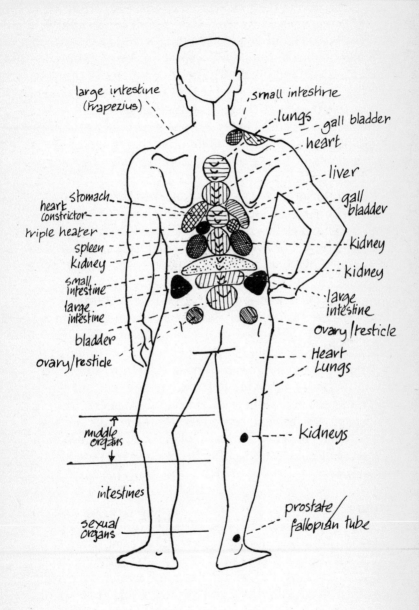

The *hara* is termed the 'ocean of *Ki*' and reflects more the short-term or acute conditions, as it is located in the more yin soft area of the body. We tend to protect this area both physically and emotionally. The muscle and skin tone are a good indicator of the person's lifestyle. Many people suffer bloating and tension in the abdomen and cannot be touched in this area during the first treatment. Because of its location it reflects the state of the digestive and reproductive organs. This is also the area of our primal intuition and instinct; you might often hear people say they had a 'gut' feeling about something which had no other logical explanation.

The posterior torso can be divided into three main areas, reflecting the long-term condition of various organs. Because the back is a more solid and well-protected area, changes here occur over a longer period. It is considered to be a more yang, harder area; if a brick was thrown at you you would normally turn your back to present the most protected side. Therefore it in turn reflects conditions of a more chronic nature which have been building up over a lengthy period. The upper third, from the shoulder level to the end of the shoulder blades, reflects the condition of the heart, lungs and diaphragm. The middle third shows the middle organs – the liver, gallbladder, stomach, spleen and pancreas and kidneys. The lower third shows the kidneys, intestines and reproductive organs' functions. Distortions, hair growth, moles, blemishes, puffiness, skin rashes or discolourations all indicate different possible imbalances.

Legs and feet

The buttocks reflect the lower digestive functions of the small intestine and the reproductive function. Loose flabby buttocks indicate weakness in the reproductive and digestive systems; the sexual libido and menstrual cycle are probably erratic. Piles and haemorrhoids are symptoms of poor digestion and eating habits as well as mental and emotional stress.

The inside area of the upper thigh should be well toned.

If there are indicators such as discolourations, flabbiness, lack of power in closing the legs, or general weakness here, then the reproductive system is over burdened and not functioning correctly. The back of the thigh also reflects the reproductive condition.

The knees show the middle organ function, as does their complementary area, the elbows. The knees generally reflect the state of the liver function, with certain variations relating to stomach and spleen also. The back of the knees reflect the condition of the kidney energy.

The calves are often tender and tense to the touch. This is an indication of an imbalanced function of the intestines. Cramping in the calves is a common problem and can be related to the generally weakened condition of the digestive function. Usually there is either an excessive intake of salt and/or sugar.

The ankles, as with the wrists, indicate the reproductive system function. The Achiles tendon should

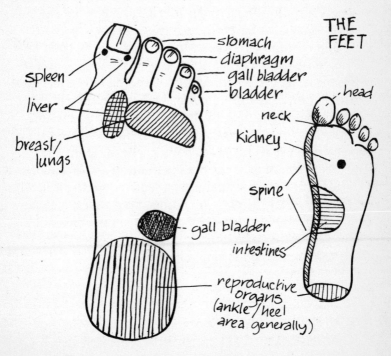

THE FEET

spleen
liver
breast/lungs

stomach
diaphragm
gall bladder
bladder

head
neck
kidney
spine

gall bladder
intestines

reproductive organs
(ankle/heel area generally)

be flexible and pain free. Puffiness and swelling of the ankles is common in menstruation, indicating blockage in the elimination function of the menstrual cycle. The outside ankle area reflects the condition of the testicles and ovaries, and pain or discolouration here show imbalances. The inside ankle area shows the condition of the uterus and prostate.

The toes have the leg meridians beginning or ending in them. The meridians in the dorsal aspect of the feet are the liver, spleen, stomach, gallbladder and bladder. The kidney is found in the underfoot area. Like the hands, tension is often held in the feet and they need to be cared for with regular massage. It is always good to walk around barefoot outside occasionally so that the feet can receive some much-needed stimulation. They are always cushioned inside shoes and receive little stimulation this way.

Bo and Yu points

In addition to the above diagnostic areas there are some specific *tsubo* used for both diagnosis and treatment of acute and chronic conditions. In the front of the body are certain *tsubo* known as alarm points and called *bo* points in Japanese. These are indicators of more acute conditions relating to the 12 organ functions and specifically to the corresponding meridian. In the back, down the sides of the spinal column, there are other special *tsubo* known as associated effect points or *yu* points. These reflect the longer term function of the organs themselves. When one of these points becomes painful or sensitive to the touch it is telling you that the corresponding organ energy needs rebalancing. The acute nature of the *bo* points means that these will change more rapidly than the *yu* points which have taken longer to develop abnormalities.

Tongue diagnosis

Because the therapist will not make his or her final diagnosis on any one feature alone, it is sometimes necessary to confirm the diagnosis with a slightly different approach.

As with the face, specific areas of the tongue reflect the functions of the various organs of the body. The shape of the tongue, whether it is long and sharp ended or more squat and rounded, give constitutional facts about the patient. The fact that your tongue may be heavily coated with white or yellow mucus also tells the therapist about your condition.

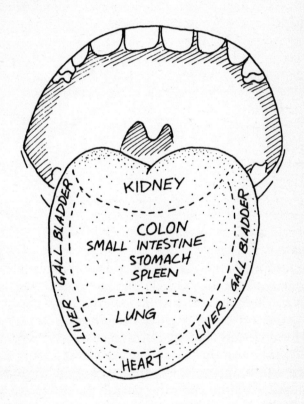

Eye diagnosis

The eyes are thought of as the 'windows to the soul'. Sparkly clear eyes reflect a healthy condition; dull lacklustre eyes indicate poor health. The eyes also reveal the general condition of the liver function. Mucus discharges in the eyes show congestion in the organs, due to fat retention and poor elimination of waste. The sclera or white of the eye is like a map of the whole body and different sections show the condition of corresponding organs.

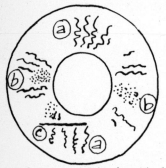

a - Expanded blood capillaries
b - White mucus patches
c - Straight long red line

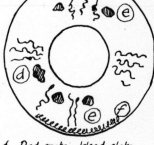

d - Red spots - blood clots
e - Dark spots
f - Mucus under the eyeball

THE HEALING EXPERIENCE

It is interesting to take an objective view of the healing phenomena which take place after shiatsu or treatment with other therapies which work on initiating a change or boost in the body's self-healing mechanism.

We have already seen that symptoms merely reflect the cause elsewhere in the body – the exterior is a reflection of the interior. Symptoms affect the organs from the more vital to the less vital, and disappear in the reverse order to which they appeared. However, symptoms often seemingly disappear, only to recur during therapy as an apparent adverse reaction. This is simply the body trying to heal itself and reverse the process by eliminating from inside to outside. Patients may break out in rashes or boils in some circumstances, as the previously locked-in toxins begin to discharge themselves from the body.

It is therefore important to keep such events in perspective. It may be temporarily uncomfortable, but it is necessary in order to relieve the problem finally. Healing yourself and maintaining good health needs to be a conscious decision and should go on for the rest of your life.

5

THE FIVE TRANSFORMATIONS OF ENERGY

The principles of Oriental medicine are based in the study of nature and natural phenomena. Yin and yang describe the movement of energy vibration as it moves upwards and outwards or downwards and inwards. These terms can be used to describe the physical structure of tangible objects as well as tendencies in the movement of the energy needed to create a particular structure. They can also be used to describe a state of mind or personality. You probably know the yin type person who is easy-going, calm to the point of docility and very much a thinker, particularly on a spiritual level. Conversely, the yang type person is very active, to the point of hypertension, tends to be impatient and is usually in a hurry about life in general.

Energy movement has many different faces. Everything changes, nothing remains the same forever. This is obvious in animate objects such as ourselves. We are born, we mature, then we die. This is the cycle of life and is simply energy changing its form. But even inanimate objects such as buildings change their form with time. Try and think of something that doesn't change. Very difficult. Even our thoughts are energetic waves which have a beginning, maturity and an end. Many philosophies such as Buddhism and Taoism concentrate on this concept of the constant movement of energy.

SEASONS OF THE YEAR

Different times of the year have different phases of energy movement predominating. During the spring your vigour is awakened after the hibernation phase of winter. In summer your energy rises and you are generally more physically active and feel more 'alive'. This energetic high begins to subside in the late summer as you start planning for the winter months and holidays to get away from the cold. Autumn is the settling-down period, before the coming of the coldness of winter again.

This is of course a never-ending cycle and greatly affects your body rhythms and general energy. You've probably noticed a pattern regarding colds or flu that you get in the same period each year. Do you always get depressed in the winter, when going out seems not worth the effort? Many people would prefer to miss the winter completely and hibernate until it's all over.

The seasons have their own natures and the downwards or yang energy movement of winter is opposite to that of the more yin upwards movement of summer. Think about the sap in the trees. During the spring and summer the sap rises to nurture new life in the leaves; during autumn and winter the sap has fallen and the leaves also fall.

THE SEASONAL DAY

Each day reflects the same seasonal changes that occur in the yearly cycle. Springtime is the period from early predawn to mid-morning; high summer is the mid-morning through to noon; late summer is the middle afternoon; autumn is the late afternoon to early evening – many people find this the most tiring time of day as the energetic direction changes; winter is the full night.

Should you have a noticeable low ebb in your energy level during a particular part of the day then the related organ imbalance can be determined. Organ functions relate to different seasons, as follows:

- Spring – liver and gallbladder.
- High summer – heart, small intestine, heart constrictor and triple warmer.

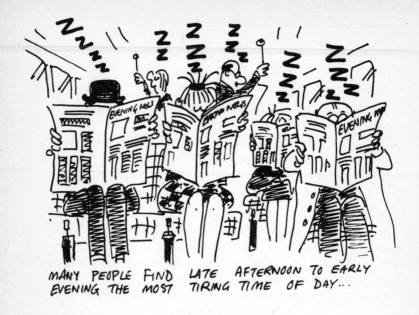

MANY PEOPLE FIND LATE AFTERNOON TO EARLY EVENING THE MOST TIRING TIME OF DAY...

- Late summer – stomach, spleen and pancreas.
- Autumn – lung and large intestine.
- Winter – bladder and kidney.

KO AND *SHEN* CYCLES

It is considered that the different meridian energies interact with one another in a supporting or nourishing cycle known as the *shen* cycle, and in a restricting or inhibiting cycle known as the *ko* cycle. The five transformations, or elements as they are sometimes called, are wood, fire, soil, metal and water. These natural elements interact in a creative cycle of complementary opposites, energetic movements which have the effect of creating and maintaining balance in all things. Each element is represented in a yin and yang organ, as everything in nature must have interacting energies; nothing is neuter, everything has some aspect of its opposite.

The more solid structured yang organs are the liver, lungs, spleen/pancreas, kidneys, heart constrictor and

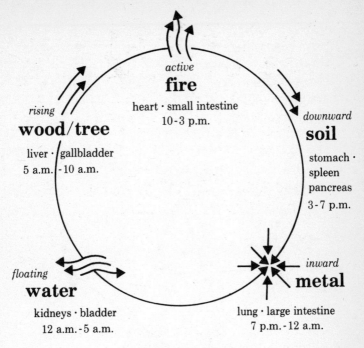

SHEN CYCLE

heart. These organs primarily control the internal functions. The more hollow yin organs are the large intestine, small intestine, stomach, bladder, gallbladder and triple heater. These organs primarily control the external functions, things affecting the body from the outside.

The elements are created and destroyed according to the law of cyclical change. The creative *shen* cycle acts as follows:

- Wood acts as fuel for fire.
- Fire generates heat to create the ash of soil.
- Soil nurtures the growth of metal.
- Metal contains the body of water.
- Water feeds and nourishes wood.

The destructive *ko* cycle acts as follows:

- Wood covers the soil.
- Soil covers or fills water.
- Water puts out fire.
- Fire melts metal.
- Metal cuts wood.

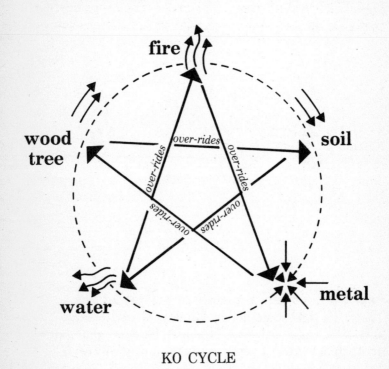

KO CYCLE

DIAGNOSIS AND TREATMENT

The five transformations are particularly useful as a diagnostic tool for determining energy imbalances through observation. Many personality factors and habits can be placed into the various categories of the elements. Then, once the imbalance is understood, the therapist is able to design a specific treatment by using the creative or destructive cycle to create balance. For example, if there is a deficiency in the water element, this energy may be boosted by attention to the metal element in the *shen* cycle. Further, the destructive overriding nature of soil may be blocking the energy flow, and here further attention may be needed. Also if the fire organs are demanding energetic attention, this may be drawing on an already low water energy. The experienced therapist has to decide the best course of action in the circumstances.

Five transformations table

Elements	Wood	Fire
Viscera	Liver	Heart
		Heart constrictor
Bowels	Gallbladder	Small intestine
		Triple warmer
Functions	Organisation	Communication
		Awareness
	Decision	Regulation
Seasons	Spring	Summer
Seasonal time of day	5am–10am	10am–3pm
Chinese clock	11pm–3am	11am–3pm (HT/SI*)
		7pm–11pm (HC/TH*)
Directions	East	South
Weather	Dry/crisp	Fog/mist
External injuring conditions	Wind	Heat
Controls on anatomy	Muscles	Arteries
	Ligaments	Circulation
	Joints	
Fluid secretions	Tears	Sweat
Body areas	Joints	Between scapulars
	Right shoulder	Chest
	Knees	
Creativity	Inspiration	Aspiration
Voice type	Shouting	Laughing
Senses	Sight	Speech
Sense organ	Eyes	Tongue
Emotions		
Negative	Anger	Excitable
	Impatience	Nervous
Positive	Patience	Joyous
	Humour	Calmness
Abnormal colour	Green	Red
	Yellow	Purple
Nurturing foods	Wheat	Corn
	Leafy green vegetables	Round leafy vegetables
Taste	Sour	Bitter
System control	Muscular	Circulatory
	Endocrine	Emotions
	Digestive	

* Heart/small intestine

* Heart constrictor/triple heater

Soil	Metal	Water
Spleen/pancreas	Lungs	Kidneys
Stomach	Large intestine	Bladder
Transformation	Exchange	Purification
Assimilation	Transmission	Vitality
	Interpretation	
Late summer	Autumn	Winter
3pm–7pm	7pm–12am	12am–5am
7am–11am	3am–7am	3pm–7pm
Equator	West	North
Mellow	Snow	Frost/ice
Humidity	Cold	Dryness
Flesh	Skin	Bones
Immune system	Membranes	Nails
		Hair
Saliva	Mucus	Urine
Knees	Shoulders	Ankles
Elbows	Abdomen	Wrists
Mid back	Chest	Buttocks
Intellect	Dominance	Will
Singing	Weeping	Groaning
Taste	Smell	Hearing
Mouth	Nose	Ears
Cynical	Grief	Fear
Jealous	Depression	Insecure
Compassion	Positive	Courage
Grounded	Stability	Confidence
Brown	White	Black
Orange	Pale	Blue
Millet	Rice	Pulses
Root vegetables	Ginger	Sea vegetables
Sweet	Pungent	Salty
Lymphatic	Respiratory	Nervous
Immune	Elimination	Hormonal
Digestive		Reproduction

6
SOME SPECIFIC CONDITIONS HELPED BY SHIATSU

The types of conditions that shiatsu is successful in helping is not unlimited, and it is not magic. Most of the time it is very effective for most people; occasionally it is unsuitable and little or no improvement occurs, in which case you would be better referred to another type of therapy. Remember that shiatsu will generally improve your health and this will involve the gradual disappearance of nagging symptoms – physical, emotional and psychological.

ADDICTIONS

Addictions cover a wide variety of problems, from drug addiction to smoking, overeating and excess alcohol consumption. Stress is a common denominator in these conditions. Obviously, the length of time and seriousness of the particular problem will be a determining factor in the length of the recovery time.

There is no particular shiatsu treatment designed to make you give up, say, smoking, but what regularly occurs is that the symptom, in this case the smoking, may be controlled as the health of the patient improves.

BACKACHE

Backache, like any other symptom, may have a variety of causes. You may lift something awkwardly, receive a sudden jarring, be damaged by a blow to the back, as in a sports car accident, or, as quite often occurs, you may simply wake up one day with this problem. So, in addition to an external cause, as in the first examples, the therapist may also have to consider an internal cause, as in the last example. If your kidney function is overworked, attempting to purify large amounts of alcohol, for example, then the contributing external factor as well as the resulting damage needs to be remedied. If the muscle structure which should support your lower back is weakened then aches and pains will occur at the least provocation. Backaches are one of the most common conditions treated by shiatsu therapists, and with much success.

EMOTIONAL AND PSYCHOLOGICAL STRESS

Because shiatsu is not limited to the physical conditions alone, it is very powerful in assisting in stabilising stress-related symptoms. By looking for and dealing with both the internal and external factors involved, a subtle non-traumatic change will be encouraged.

LETHARGY

Lethargy affects almost everyone from time to time. This is usually because you have been overworking, overplaying, not eating well, not exercising, or just bored. For this symptom to occur occasionally is not unhealthy; it is your body telling you to slow down and rest for a while, to recuperate. However, if you are perpetually lethargic, then this is an indication of chronic energy blockages. Lethargy is not just physical tiredness but also a mental and emotional affliction; you are usually too depressed to do anything about being depressed. Remove the energy blockages and the factors contributing to their gradual build up, and the lethargy disappears.

Once again there are numerous factors involved and your therapist will determine which energy imbalances need to be remedied. There may also be some commonsense advice, such as reducing the intake of caffeine which attacks the adrenal glands and kidney energy, responsible for your vitality and willpower.

MIGRAINE

The migraine headache is very common these days. The medical description of this type of headache is hemicrania, a unilateral throbbing type of headache with at least three of the following features: sensory pain; photophobia, light sensitivity; nausea or vomiting; fluid retention before or during the headache; diuresis, increased urination; family history of migraine.

There are always a variety of factors which cause headaches, and the fact that these causatory factors are different for everyone is now apparent. Furthermore, the use of drug therapy only suppresses the symptoms without changing the cause. Shiatsu can be the instigator for change in these circumstances. Having a course of treatments, and following dietary and exercise advice, will have the effect of changing your mental, emotional and physical states which were previously disturbed or blocked and which allowed the migraine symptoms to occur. The emphasis is thus on you, the patient, to investigate and effect changes in your own lifestyle as a preventative measure, as well as receiving the assistance of your therapist.

PREGNANCY AND CHILDBIRTH

Pregnancy and childbirth should be the most natural series of events in a woman's life. The use of drugs and hormone therapy in pregnancy is generally not necessary in a healthy woman; these strong chemical interventions can disrupt the energetic development of the embryo. Even shiatsu, which is very subtle, should not be applied too strenuously or too frequently during the first three months. However, shiatsu is effective in encouraging a healthy and happy attitude towards being pregnant, an attitude which is sometimes lacking due to symptoms such as morning sickness, fluid retention and lethargy.

Active childbirth is now common and popular among younger parents. The effective study and application of daily exercise, breathing techniques and meditation for stress control gives you the best possible chance of having a stress-free birth. I encourage my patients to attend shiatsu sessions with their partners so that both parents are prepared for the psychological and physical demands of childbirth, this being especially helpful for first time pregnancies. Shiatsu at the birth can often eliminate the need for drugs to induce the baby, and is very helpful for labour pain relief.

REPRODUCTIVE SYSTEM PROBLEMS

The reproductive system incorporates the primary and secondary sex organs as well as the kidney and bladder purification and waste elimination functions in both males and females. Women are generally more forthcoming than men in seeking assistance in alleviating reproductive related problems. One reason for this is that women have the inbuilt monitor of the menstrual cycle to sound a warning in times of dis-ease. And even when men are aware of problems, such as impotence, premature ejaculation or discomfort in urination, they still appear to be inhibited about seeking help.

The reproductive organs function is very much affected by the supply of *ki* and blood. For circulation to be effective in the pelvic area, the pelvic diaphragm, also called the pelvic floor, must be made to move. This stimulates muscle activity and blood movement. If you do not 'move' this area, then waste products, toxins and fatty deposits settle and accumulate, like dirty water left sitting in a sink. This continuous build up of waste matter becomes harder, and unless eliminated will eventually turn into fibroids, cysts and tumours. This accumulation itself further restricts the energy flow, unless changes are made through shiatsu and the introduction of exercise and dietary changes.

Shiatsu is helpful in 'regulating' the menstrual cycle and alleviating other symptoms such as pre-menstrual tension, cramping and oedema, and is sometimes helpful in chronic infertility conditions. Male conditions, mentioned above, can also be helped greatly.

SERIOUS CHRONIC ILLNESSES

Serious and chronic illnesses such as cancer, heart disease, or AIDS are, by their very nature, more difficult to control and treat successfully. The state of degeneration and damage in each individual case will determine the relative success of shiatsu in aiding the body's natural self-healing mechanism, and the shiatsu would have to be combined with dietary and stress control exercises and other lifestyle changes to be of most benefit. In terminally ill cases the patients' enjoyment of life and attitude to their condition will be enhanced by shiatsu, and in such circumstances I would consider this a successful treatment.

SPORTS INJURIES

Many professional athletes, dancers, footballers and others involved in potentially injurious activities have regular shiatsu as a means of not only preventing injury but also improving performance. The therapist may also use other techniques such as moxibustion, the burning of a herb either in direct or indirect contact with the skin, and cupping, the use of suction instruments on the area of damage to draw out stagnation.

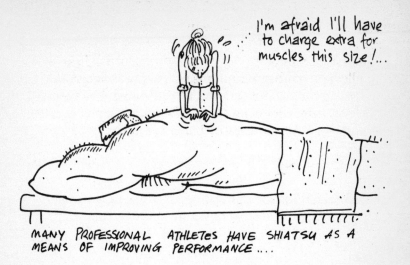

MANY PROFESSIONAL ATHLETES HAVE SHIATSU AS A MEANS OF IMPROVING PERFORMANCE....

STRUCTURAL DISORDERS

Raised shoulders, a twisted spine, restricted neck movement, twisted hips, distended or swollen organs, and damaged joints come under the category of structural distortions in shiatsu. However, the structure only changes after the energy which 'feeds' that structure has changed; therefore to correct the structure you must firstly correct the energy imbalance.

For example, you may have a damaged spinal vertebrae due to a gradual weakening of the surrounding muscle and connective tissue through lack of exercise and consequent poor *ki* and blood circulation. This resulting pain or discomfort may be alleviated by mechanical adjustment of the affected vertebrae; however, if you don't change the cause, the symptom will eventually resurface. This guideline in fact applies to any symptom; by locating the imbalanced meridian energies supplying the affected area, your therapist will be able to help your body strengthen that area so that the symptom doesn't recur.

CASE HISTORIES

Mrs C

Mrs C was 64 and suffered from chronic low back pain initiated by a sports injury in her youth. She had received a variety of therapies, including physiotherapy and osteopathy, with some improvement, but the symptoms persisted.

She had an excess in her liver energy and a deficiency in the bladder energy. Some interesting symptoms associated with these imbalances are suppressed anger and fearfulness. There were various other structural distortions adding to her problem. Her main regret was that she could no longer maintain her garden, which she enjoyed immensely. This frustration of course created a vicious circle, adding to her anger.

After a course of treatments, which involved dietary and exercise recommendations, her general flexibility improved, to the degree that she was able to commence gardening again. Consequently much of her anger and frustration disappeared, and her well-being improved greatly. She was a very satisfying case to work with.

Many elderly people come to the conclusion that they simply cannot do the physical things they used to enjoy because of their age. I have seen many of these same people delighted to be able to take up walking or gardening again after years of being unable to.

Ms D

Ms D came to see me suffering from fatigue brought about by running a very successful and growing business. She had acute neck and shoulder tension, combined with skin rashes and tightness in the chest, diarrhoea and irregular menstruation. Emotionally she was depressed, irritable, easily angered and finding her relationship stressful. The physical symptoms were the first to recede, as the emotional situation was very much related to the pressures of work and she had to sort out how to handle this stress; everyone lives under stress, some people simply handling it much better than others.

She had a deficiency in the lung energy, which was responsible for the depression. There was also a great deal of fear about her own ability to be successful, and difficulty with her self-confidence. Here her liver excess of energy was useful, as this helped her planning and organisational skills.

After a series of treatments her physical appearance changed greatly as the stress seemingly disappeared. Of course, the stress of the job was still prevalent but because she felt stronger about herself emotionally she was no longer adversely affected by it.

Mr I

Mr I was 32, self-employed and was having difficulties in his relationship, with physical symptoms of left side tension, general lethargy and lack of sexual libido. He always felt restless and held much tension in his chest. The shoulders and low back were a chronic problem. Emotionally he was lacking confidence in himself and his relationship.

After several treatments his sense of well-being resurfaced and his physical symptoms gradually disappeared. The relationship difficulties were seen in a different perspective and he and his partner subsequently had a baby. His was a case not of having any particular serious deficiency or excess of energy, but more a problem of how his energy was being distributed in the body. He was like a jigsaw puzzle; he had all the right energetic pieces but they were not in the correct places.

Mr S

Mr S had a history of back pains, and came to see me after injuring himself playing squash. Other physical symptoms involved were constipation and neck tension. He was also suffering from lethargy and depression. In his case, the chronic nature of the back weakness came from a history of digestive problems including intestinal viruses from various travels; the large intestine energy gives support, particularly to the area of lumbar vertebrae four and five, and this was the focal point of discomfort.

By giving him shiatsu, and with particular emphasis on dietary advice, his condition gradually improved. The shiatsu gave him immediate pain relief for the sciatica, but he had to strengthen his large intestine energy in general to maintain a strong back. His constipation cleared and so did emotional aspects involved with constipation, such as holding onto emotions; like the physical phenomenon of holding on to the body's waste matter, he was not expressing his emotions adequately. His overall flexibility improved, and regular exercise and a better diet kept his back in good condition.

Ms M

Ms M was 36 and had a long history of menstrual irregularities and related problems. She originally started taking the contraceptive pill to regulate her periods and, as often occurs, she found herself without any periods when she finally stopped taking the pill. She wanted to become pregnant but wasn't able to conceive. Other symptoms involved were indigestion, constipation, neck and shoulder tension and lower backache. She did little exercise and did not eat well. She felt a lot of anger in general and was easily irritated and always impatient.

The energy controlling the reproductive system was imbalanced. She had a deficiency in her bladder and spleen meridians and excess in the liver. Physically her right kidney, which controls the more yin energy movement, was congested and tight. Her abdomen was bloated and she had regular flatulence.

After three treatments and dietary and exercise implementation her digestive problems improved. Once the digestion had improved, her elimination of excess meant she had less congestion in her reproductive organs.

After about six months her periods returned and she eventually became pregnant. Her reproductive system had simply been clogged up through a combination of poor digestion caused by an inadequate diet and stress, together with a lack of abdominal exercise to help the circulation and elimination processes.

7
WHAT DOES A TREATMENT INVOLVE?

A shiatsu session usually lasts about one hour and the treatment itself is anywhere between 35 and 50 minutes.

In your first session your therapist will spend time obtaining information about you, in order to make up your case history. This is a confidential record of your personal details, symptoms, diagnostic details and treatments given. The duration of this question/answer period differs from therapist to therapist. The types of questions involved refer to your health history – injuries sustained, surgical history, any major illnesses such as diabetes, hepatitis, malaria, spinal injuries, and other stress-related illnesses. You will probably also be asked questions about your diet, exercise routine and stress areas of your life.

Many common problems such as backache may be caused by your occupational sitting position, for example, and may be alleviated through changes in the type of office furniture used and/or specific exercises to relieve the problem. A woman may simply have to throw away her high heel shoes to lessen greatly her chronic backache or shoulder tension; high heels cause excessive stress and can create distortion of the musculoskeletal system.

Question diagnosis is very important, but, as seen in Chapter 4, it is only one of a number of types of diagnosis used in deciding the outline of the treatment best suited to the patient. Each treatment is unique in that it is specifically designed to suit the needs of the patient whose symptoms, and background to those symptoms, are

unique to that person. The other types of diagnosis used
are as follows:

- Visual – the facial diagnostic areas, the posture,
  movement, skin colour and reactions are some of the
  features observed.
- Touch – feeling body, muscle and skin tone, testing
  mobility and feeling the meridians for areas of excess
  or deficiency.
- Senses – a particular odour, breathing sound or voice
  quality may attract the therapist's attention indicating
  an imbalance in certain organs.
- Intuition – the therapist's experience may indicate
  another possible problem which requires investigation,
  for example, some past emotional trauma causing
  energy blockages.

Once the therapist has made a composite diagnosis,
based on all the information presented, the treatment will
begin.

Touch is the most important and essential aspect of
shiatsu. Touch tells the therapist things about the patient
which questions do not necessarily reveal. Therefore, the
diagnosis continues throughout the whole treatment and
the therapist is always gathering new information about
the patient.

The physical examination

Besides looking at your face and skin condition there will
be other physical examinations. It is likely you may be
asked to walk up and down the room. This discloses
bilateral imbalances, as well as any distortions in the
major joint areas such as hips and shoulders. Flexibility
assessment indicates the state of muscle and meridian
tone. For example, you may be asked if you can still touch
your toes (this will improve after shiatsu); as you stretch
to touch your toes your, torso may pull to one side or the
other, indicating imbalances in the upper and lower torso
and leg meridians.

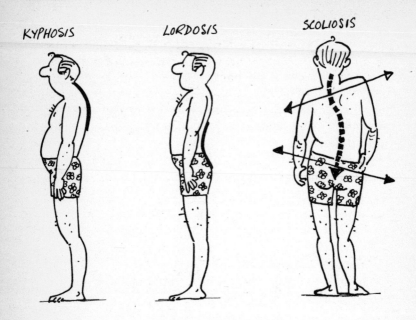

KYPHOSIS   LORDOSIS   SCOLIOSIS

Distortions of the spine

HOW MANY TREATMENTS DO I NEED?

Shiatsu is a very powerful and effective therapy. However, it is not magic and problems which have maybe taken years to develop cannot be alleviated in one treatment. That frozen shoulder or menstrual irregularity didn't just happen overnight, and it will therefore take time and effort on your part to create an improvement.

A course of treatments usually involves five to seven treatments, preferably at weekly or sometimes shorter intervals. Some people make big changes in this time and don't require more, while others may need a longer course of treatment. In either situation, it must be remembered that shiatsu is also good preventative therapy, aiding the maintenance of good health, and I usually recommend that patients have further treatments every one or two months for their general health.

WHAT TO WEAR

The patient is clothed for the treatment, although the therapist will at some stage expose various parts of the body, such as the limbs, back, ankles and abdomen, to check for skin discolourations, moles, blemishes and tone. Because the treatment may involve stretching positions and some teaching of remedial exercises, it is necessary to wear loose comfortable clothing such as a tracksuit or lightweight summer cotton clothing. Cotton material is preferable because it creates little change in the body's *ki*, whereas synthetic materials make a static electricity disturbance.

AVOID A FULL STOMACH

Some methods of diagnosis and treatment involve palpitation of the abdomen. If you have just eaten, your abdomen will feel uncomfortable when touched and the digestion process will draw energy to the abdomen distorting the true diagnostic picture. It is best not to eat for a period of at least three hours prior to a treatment. It is also suggested that patients refrain from consuming alcohol on the day of treatment – there should be as little outside disturbance as possible to maintain the balancing effects of the treatment.

ARE THERE ANY INSTRUMENTS USED?

In most cases the therapist's natural tools, his or her hands, are all that is necessary. Occasionally, the use of other therapies may be incorporated into the treatment.

Moxa

This is a combustion-type technique which involves the application of heat. Moxa is a Chinese herb derived from the mugwort plant. Moxa burned on the skin at the location of a *tsubo* will stimulate the release of energetic blockages, the essence of the herb being absorbed into the system through the skin. This type of treatment helps improve the patient's resistance to disease and in treating specific conditions.

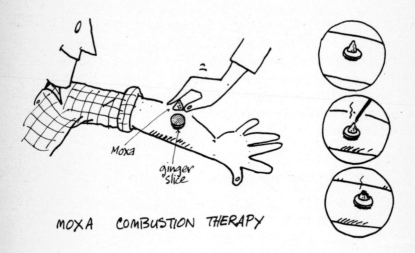

MOXA COMBUSTION THERAPY

There are different applications of this therapy. The moxa may be ignited directly on the skin surface. It may also be placed on a thin sliver of ginger which is between it and the skin, or a moxa stick may be used which is held away from the skin above the *tsubo*.

Cupping

This involves the application of suction to specific areas of injury or excess energy stagnation. Various-sized glass or plastic cups are placed on the skin surface and suction is created, either by using a flame inside the cup to use up

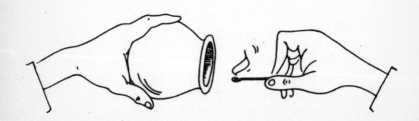

the oxygen or by the use of a hand pump. The skin surface inside the cup raises dramatically, drawing energy and sedating the area. This is very useful in sports injuries, as well as releasing those tightly knotted areas of tension found throughout the body.

AFTER EFFECTS OF SHIATSU

This differs greatly from person to person, depending on their state of health and symptoms. If a patient hasn't had any form of physical therapy previously and is unfit, the effects may be dramatic. With a regular recipient of shiatsu, who is fit, the changes will be deeper and more subtle. Basically, in the latter case there is less need for change, while in the former case the patient may actually feel slightly worse the following day. Some people even feel flu-like symptoms, aches and pains, or headaches after the first treatment. Fortunately, this lessens with each subsequent treatment. These apparent adverse after effects are the natural process of the body making an attempt to correct its own condition, commonly referred to as a healing crisis. Some things have to get worse before they can get better, and the patient usually feels much improved after a short time.

The aim of receiving shiatsu will obviously be to improve your state of well-being and to relieve symptoms. Shiatsu generally improves the skin tone, relaxes and increases muscle flexibility, heightens nervous system responses and improves your reaction time, improves your mental clarity and aids concentration, strengthens the bones and ligaments, strengthens the digestive and circulatory systems, and relieves your stressed condition, giving you a better sense of well-being and direction in life.

RECOMMENDATIONS

Your therapist may give you advice so that you can help improve your health at home as well as coming for treatments; your self-responsibility is an important factor

in achieving and maintaining good health. This advice
may take the form of simple dietary recommendations,
such as reducing or avoiding harmful stimulants like
caffeine and sugar. You may also be shown simple
corrective exercises to stretch and unblock the meridian
energy flow. It is important to follow this advice to obtain
the best results from your treatments. If deemed
necessary, you may be advised to consult another
therapist such as a cranial osteopath, acupuncturist,
herbalist, homeopath, counsellor or GP, in addition to
your shiatsu therapist, if your recovery will be assisted in
this way.

Self treatments

A general health enhancing system know as *do-in* may be
taught to you (for more details about *do-in* see Chapter 8).
There are also many simple home treatments that you will

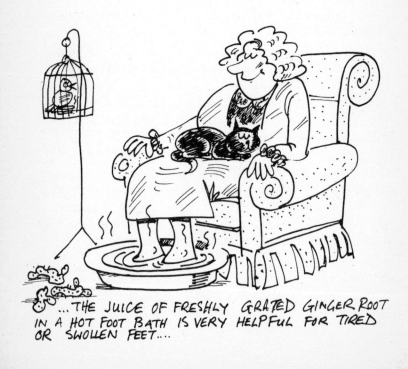

...THE JUICE OF FRESHLY GRATED GINGER ROOT
IN A HOT FOOT BATH IS VERY HELPFUL FOR TIRED
OR SWOLLEN FEET....

find easy and beneficial to perform; for example, the juice of freshly grated ginger root in a hot foot bath is very helpful for tired or swollen feet and generally improves circulation. The use of various compresses or poultices may be suggested, to assist in the relief of certain problems such as skin rashes, headaches, low energy, sinus congestion.

HOW MUCH DO I PAY

The fee for shiatsu varies, the average usually being around £15 to £25 per session (1989). Currently, shiatsu is not yet available on the National Health Service, except in a few locations.

8
TAKING CARE OF YOURSELF

Modern Western society no longer places emphasis on physical fitness and ability. Anyone who does daily exercise and generally watches their own health is often referred to as a health nut or fitness fanatic, in a begrudgingly envious but derogatory fashion. Much emphasis is placed on developing the mind to cope with the intellectual and economic demands of the modern lifestyle; children are pressured into striving for higher and higher academic achievements, with the threat of unemployment or a mundane existence if they don't have a degree or some other qualification. As with every other situation, this has both positive and negative attributes. Not enough concern is given to strengthening the body through regular daily exercise; the psychological discipline of doing and enjoying exercise is rapidly disappearing in our younger generation, and is nearly lost in their parental age group.

This dramatic change has mainly taken place in the last century, and certainly since the industrial revolution, when the agrarian society moved aside for technology. More intellectual and less physical work evolved. Cardiovascular exercise – exercise which increases the heart beat, strengthening the heart pump – became less prominent in daily work.

Today, ironically, thousands of people in the West are following centuries old Eastern traditions, studying yoga, *t'ai chi* and *do-in*, for example, in order to achieve a calm and peaceful mind and a strong physical body. However, although these exercise techniques have both physical and spiritual benefits, they alone are not enough to maintain a healthy mind, body and spirit. We tend to congratulate ourselves because we have done half an hour of *tai chi* or yoga each day; these 'forms', as they are called, calm the mind, breathing and heart rate, which is undoubtedly very important. However, we forget that the origins of these exercises come from the East where millions of people have practised them daily as part of their working day. The average Chinese practising his or her *t'ai chi* probably does so before or after a hard day of physical labour which fulfils the cardiovascular requirement for daily exercise. Here in the West, the majority don't usually do any physical labour.

Therefore, as well as our Oriental exercises, we also need to provide ourselves with some cardiovascular stimulation. You can do this through a wide variety of exercises – walking, swimming, cycling, running, tennis, golf, gardening, dancing, to name but a few. I generally don't recommend people to take up 'aerobics' type exercise unless they are already fit and can be certain of an experienced teacher; many injuries occur in aerobics when people push themselves too far too soon and overstretch muscles, ligaments and tendons.

DO-IN

Besides attending regular shiatsu sessions you need to make an effort to improve your health through self exercise. Self-responsibility is all important in making substantial and positive changes towards a healthier happier lifestyle. There is a unique system of Oriental exercises designed for this purpose, called *do-in* in Japanese. *Do-in* is a form of self-massage therapy based on stimulating the meridian system of the body.

Do-in has been used as part of Oriental medicine for many thousands of years and has continually adapted to suit the needs of modern society. It involves the enhancement of your well-being through a series of exercises including breathing, stretching, percussion, pressure application, corrective exercises and meditation.

By performing your *do-in* exercises daily you will notice great improvement in your flexibility, skin and muscle tone, inner calmness, mental clarity, circulation and emotional stability, as well as the reduction of general aches and pains, including those associated with arthritis and rheumatism.

BREATHING

Not enough emphasis is ever placed on the importance of breathing to reduce stress and improve the physical, emotional and psychological condition. The autonomic nervous system is positively stimulated by the proper use of controlled breathing. What happens to your breathing when you get angry? It becomes shallow and rapid, until the anger subsides. This is because the sympathetic branch of the autonomic nervous system has become dominant; more carbon dioxide is released into the blood stream and thinking becomes impaired.

You may have been told to breathe deeply when you feel anger, as this calms you down. Deeper breathing stimulates the parasympathetic branch of the autonomic nervous system. When this branch is dominant the heart beat and breathing slows and a sense of calm prevails; there is an increase in the amount of oxygen released into the bloodstream. By controlling the breathing through special exercise you will be able to self-induce a more relaxed and calm state of body and mind.

EXERCISES TO RELIEVE STRESS

Try this breathing exercise any time you feel stressed, as well as when you first wake in the morning and last thing at night.
- Sit in a straight-backed chair with both feet flat on the floor in front of you. Straighten your spine and tuck your chin towards your chest without straining. Place your hands in your lap, the left hand resting lightly in the right and the thumbs touching.

- Close your mouth and eyes and concentrate on the breath moving through the nostrils. After several breaths focus your concentration into your abdomen, particularly the area between the navel and the pubic bone. This is called *tan den* and is thought of as the 'ocean of *ki*'. The general area of the abdomen is called the *hara*, meaning, literally, belly.
- As you inhale through the nose, use your abdominal muscles to expand the *hara*, like a balloon filling. Try and inhale for five to seven seconds. As you exhale, still through the nose, draw in the abdominal muscles. Practise this for several breaths. You may find it difficult to begin with, but it will soon become easier and feel more natural.

If you do not wish to sit in a chair you can sit cross-legged on the floor with a pillow under your backside. The pillow is important as it allows you to retain the straight back posture without having to tense the back and abdominal muscles. The correctly maintained posture is vital to this type of breathing exercise.

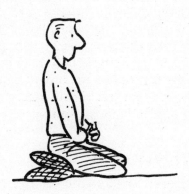

In order to calm your mind and help you to concentrate without distraction, you can use counting as one method of focusing. Practise the following procedure:
- Use the above posture. Concentrate on the intake and exhalation of breath through the nose.

- Count each combined inhalation and exhalation as one. Make a picture of a blank cinema screen in your mind's eye.
- With each breath project the numbers from one to ten in sequence in your mind; first breath combination is one, the second breath combination is two, and so on.
- Each time your concentration on the numbers strays and you think about something else, like your work or food, you have to begin counting at one again.

You will probably find that you don't often make it to ten when you practise this exercise; this doesn't matter. Try to do this exercise for ten minutes daily.

MERIDIAN STIMULATION – PERCUSSION AND STRETCHING

Stretches
This is a selection of just a few of the meridian enhancing exercises.
- Sit on the floor with your legs out in front of you. Have the ankles touching. Your torso should be straight upright. Stretch both arms above your head. Breathe in, stretch forward from the hips and touch your toes whilst exhaling. Hold the stretch for five seconds.

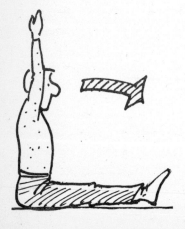
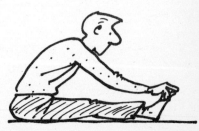

Inhale as you straighten the spine, with the arms still extended, returning to the starting position. Repeat three times. This stimulates the kidney and bladder meridians.

- Lie back, facing upwards. Have your legs outstretched and your feet about 12 inches apart, your arms by your sides, palm up. Breathe into the *hara* and follow the breathing for one minute. This is called the relaxation pose, and should be used between sets of exercises or at any time you wish to relax.

- Take a standing position with the feet shoulder-distance apart and arms by the sides. Bend the knees slightly to lower your centre of gravity. Using either hand, massage the back of the neck while the head is tilted forward at a 45 degree angle. Concentrate on loosening any tight areas.

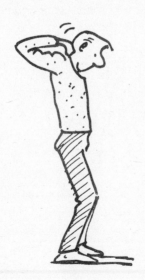

- Stand with the feet shoulder-width apart and knees straight. Place your hands behind your back and take your right thumb in your left hand. Inhale, then as you exhale bend forward from the hips, bringing the head towards the feet whilst raising your clasped hands up

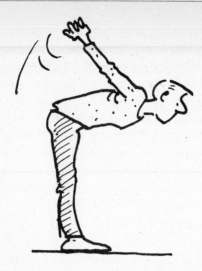

towards your head from behind. This stimulates the
lung and large intestine meridians. Repeat three times.
- Stand with the feet together, arms by the sides. Make
  a connection with the thumb and index finger on each

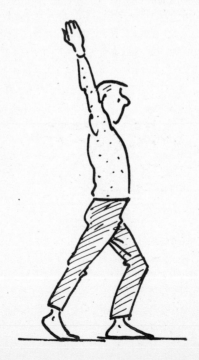

hand; this creates a circuit of energy for the respiratory system (see the diagram of lung and large intestine meridians on page 25). Inhale as you step forward with the right foot and bending at the right knee, raising the arms above your head with the upper arms close to the ears. Feel the stretch in the front of the body and the inside arms. Hold for five seconds. Exhale as you return to the original position. Repeat the exercise with the left foot forward, then repeat the whole exercise three times. This stretches the lung and stomach meridians.

- Go into the relaxation pose.
- Still lying down, spread the arms and legs as wide as is comfortably possible; relax in this position for a few moments. Inhale as you bring the legs together and draw the knees up on to the chest, wrapping the arms around the knees, the head coming up to touch the knees. Hold this position for five seconds whilst breathing normally. Exhale whilst returning to the starting position, coordinating the breath and movement so that the limbs reach the starting position simultaneously. Repeat five times. This is good for the nervous system and for general tonification.

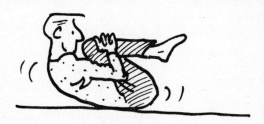

- This next exercise is good for general muscle relaxation; you will also find it useful in promoting a deeper and more relaxing sleep if done last thing at night when in bed. Lie in the relaxation pose. Focus on your abdominal breathing, feeling the rise and fall of the abdomen. Now bring your mental focus into your toes; clench the toes. Move your focus into the feet;

clench the feet, still keeping the toes clenched. Pull
your toes back towards your head, stretching the
Achilles tendon, tighten the calves; toes and feet
should still be clenched. Try and breathe as normally
as possible. Continue moving your mental focus up the
body to the knees, thighs, buttocks, abdomen, lower
back, chest, shoulders, upper back, arms, forearms;
clench the fists, the neck, tighten the facial muscles.
Your whole body should now be tensed. Breathe in,
then breathe out and totally relax all your clenched
muscles. Everything should feel relaxed. Repeat three
times.

Percussion exercises to tone up the meridians

A simple yet effective way of stimulating your own
meridian system can be performed in five minutes, once
you have practised it several times. This exercise will help
release tension and energy blockages in the meridians.

- Stand upright, with feet shoulder distance apart.
  Relax the shoulders and legs.
- Make a loose fist and wrist and, using both hands,
  gently tap the scalp to stimulate blood circulation and
  brain function. This is also helpful in preventing hair
  loss. With the tips of the fingers massage the scalp as
  if washing your hair.
- Using the palms of the hands and or the finger tips,
  rub the face vigorously. Be sure to massage the
  forehead, sides of the nose, temples, upper and lower
  jaws and jaw hinge near the ear. Brush the ears until
  they feel hot.
- Using the loosely clenched fists, tap down the back
  and sides of the neck, then squeeze and massage the
  neck muscles and the muscles in the top of the
  shoulder. This shoulder and neck area retains a lot of
  tension and is often related to overeating and
  overworking.
- Using the left hand to support the right elbow, tap
  across the top of the left shoulder with your right
  hand, and up and down the left side of your back as

far as you can reach. Release the elbow, then tap from
the left shoulder to the hand along the inside part of
the arm. Now tap from the hand back up to the left
shoulder along the outside of the arm. Repeat three
times.

- Working on the left hand, rotate each finger by holding
  it between the right index finger and thumb.
- Do the previous two exercises on your right shoulder,
  arm and hand.
- Tap across the chest above and around the breasts
  and across the ribs. Massage the breasts; this is
  particularly useful in the case of menstrual-related
  problems and throughout pregnancy.
- Place one hand on top of the other and make a circular
  motion around the abdomen in a clockwise direction,
  down the left and up the right side. Continue for about
  30 seconds.
- Using the back of your hands vigorously rub your
  lower back from as high up the back as possible to the
  buttocks. Tap the buttocks with loose fists. This
  stimulates the lower digestive and reproductive
  systems.
- With the back of your open hand tap the sacrum, the
  bony plate at the base of the spine. This will stimulate
  the central nervous system. Tapping the tail bone
  gently has the effect of clearing the sinuses.
- Have the legs about three feet apart while still
  standing. Keep the knees locked and start tapping
  down the outside of both legs with loose fists. Go from
  the sides of the buttocks to the ankle. Then tap up the
  inside of the legs from the ankle to the groin. Repeat
  three times.
- Sit on the floor. Concentrating on one foot at a time,
  use your closed fist to 'knuckle' the sole. Massage
  between the bones on the front of the foot with the tips
  of the fingers. As you did with the fingers, rotate and
  massage each toe to stimulate the energy and blood
  flow. The leg meridian pathways can all be found in
  the feet, so attention given to this area is very

beneficial, particularly if you suffer from poor
circulation or arthritis.

As stated earlier, this programme will probably take 15
minutes to begin with, but as you gain experience you can
do it in five minutes. Of course, doing the exercise in as
short a time as possible is not necessarily the best
approach. Try and allow 20 minutes to give yourself a
little caring attention; your mind and body will appreciate
it.

DIET AND YOUR HEALTH

Of course, exercise alone cannot maintain a healthy state.
The two ways in which we revitalise our *ki* is through
respiration and nutrition. Our food is our fuel, and the
better the quality of fuel the greater will be your
performance. The Second World War was the real start of
processed food production in large quantity. Ever since
then food manufacturers have striven to make eating as
simple and work free as possible. Chemicals added to
growing crops and chemicals and preservatives in food
processing have all been a contributing factor in the
general decline of our health. The average life expectancy
may have increased, but what about the actual quality of
that life, surviving on drugs and surgery as symptomatic
treatment?

A balanced diet simply means:

- Avoid extremes of poor quality foods such as
  processed and chemicalised foods.
- Too much fatty acid or saturated fats are consumed in
  the form of meat and dairy products; these are major
  contributing factors in heart disease and other
  degenerative diseases such as cancer.
- You should try to eat fresh vegetables and fruit
  products daily, together with a staple of whole cereal
  grains such as brown rice, millet, barley or corn.
- White meat fish is less fatty and usually provides good
  nourishment, unless it comes from a particularly
  polluted area; it is always worthwhile checking its
  source.

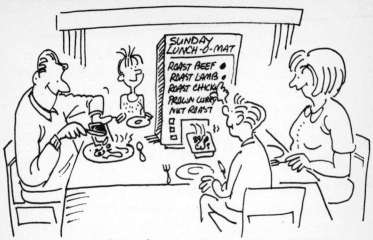

A BALANCED DIET SIMPLY MEANS : AVOID EXTREMES
OF POOR QUALITY FOODS SUCH AS PROCESSED AND
CHEMICALISED FOODS ....

If your main emphasis is on eating wholefoods and
preferably organic fruit and vegetables, this will be a good
start. More and more major supermarkets are stocking
wholefoods and organic vegetables; if enough people
enquire, then that demand will be met for purely
economic if not ideological reasons.

Now is the time to change your ideas about your own
health. You need to begin a daily routine of exercise and
healthier eating. However, it is important to approach
these changes slowly and make a comfortable transition
from one approach to the other. The combination of better
food and regular exercise will make you feel more alive
and aware of your own body. An important suggestion is
to chew your food slowly and as many as 50 times per
mouthful, as this is the first stage of digestion. This will
relieve many digestive related problems. Eating should be
meditative and not rushed, if for no other reason than to
enjoy the true taste of what you are eating. Many cases of
tightness in the neck and shoulders – a diagnostic area for
digestive disorders – can be greatly relieved by giving your
eating more time and concentration.

How does my diet affect my children's health?

It has recently been discovered that heart disease can actually begin in children from the age of five or six onwards. This is a frightening prospect. How can a healthy child develop potential heart problems so young? But think about it. If you as a parent live a lifestyle which has resulted in your own heart becoming weak, then those very same dietary and emotional habits which influenced your own heart will probably be followed by your offspring.

It is vitally important for a mother during pregnancy to eat cleanly and avoid alcohol and cigarettes, as this has been shown to affect the health of the new-born child. Whilst breastfeeding you should remember that everything you consume becomes food for your baby. This is a very big responsibility.

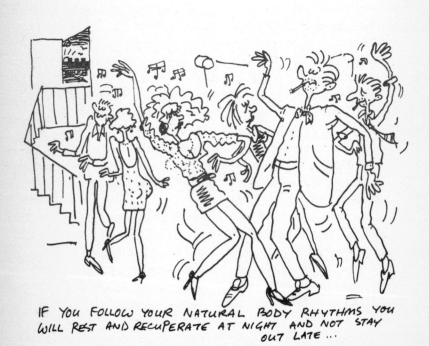

IF YOU FOLLOW YOUR NATURAL BODY RHYTHMS YOU WILL REST AND RECUPERATE AT NIGHT AND NOT STAY OUT LATE...

SLEEP

Too much work and exercise will tire you out; a balance needs to be maintained. Try and retire before midnight and awake at dawn for the most restful and refreshing sleep. During the night the body moves frequently in an attempt to manipulate itself to correct any distortions brought about by the day's activities. Thinking of the 24-hour cycle as reflecting the four seasons of the year, it is easy to understand that night is the equivalent of winter; it is dark and there is the need to be warm, to be well-fed, to hibernate. If you follow your natural body rhythms, which follow these same seasonal changes, then you will rest and recuperate at night and not stay out late.

This is, of course, a general guideline, and doesn't mean you can't go out occasionally. Leisure time is as important as sleep. Just keep the correct balance, for your own condition. The deep sleep exercise on page 97 and the breathing exercise are helpful for an undisturbed sleep.

USEFUL ADDRESSES

HOW DO I FIND A THERAPIST?

There is a governing body for shiatsu therapists, called the Shiatsu Society, which maintains a list of registered therapists in Great Britain who are subject to a code of ethics and practice. Duly qualified therapists will have the letters MRSS after their name, denoting Member of the Register of the Shiatsu Society. The list of therapists may be obtained from the following address:

The Shiatsu Society
19 Langside Park
Kilbarchan
Renfrewshire PA10 2EP
Scotland
05057 4657

Some clinics in London
Community Health Foundation
188 Old Street
London EC1
01-251 4076

Natureworks
16 Balderton Street
London W1
01-355 4036

HOW CAN I STUDY SHIATSU?

Once again, the Shiatsu Society provides information about courses in Great Britain. At present there are several major colleges offering courses in Shiatsu in this country.

British School of Shiatsu-Do
East West Centre
188 Old Street
London EC1V 9BP
01-251 0831

The British School of Shiatsu-Do has internationally
affiliated schools in Switzerland and the United States.

UK affiliated schools of the British School of Shiatsu-Do
The Bristol School of Shiatsu
18 Lilymead Avenue
Knowle
Bristol BS4 2BX
0272 772809

The East Anglia School of Shiatsu
2 Capondale Cottages
New Lane
Holbrook
Ipswich
Suffolk IP9 2RB
0473 328 061

Other colleges
The European School of Shiatsu
6 Palace Gate
Kensington Gardens
London W8

Healing-Shiatsu Education Centre
The Orchard
Lower Maescod
Hereford HR2 0HP
087 387 207

The Heart of England Shiatsu School
238 Cubbington Road
Lillington
Leamington Spa
Warwickshire
0926 881615

The Shiatsu College
20a Lower Goat Lane
Norwich NR2 1EL
0603 632555

OTHER CENTRES FOR INFORMATION

Community Health Foundation
188 Old Street
London EC1V 9BP
01-251 4076
Provides a wide range of facilities for introductory courses
in complementary medicine, including shiatsu and
macrobiotics.

The Institute for Complementary Medicine
21 Portland Place
London W1N 3AF
01-636 9543
Provides an information service for the public and
professionals on how to find registered practitioners and
organisations.

FURTHER READING

Here is a suggested reading list for books about shiatsu and Oriental medicine.

Shiatsu Practitioners Manual, Saul Goodman, Langhorne PA, United States – INFI-TECH 1986.

Zen Shiatsu, Shizuto Masunaga and Wataru Ohashi, Japan Publications, Tokyo, 1977.

Zen Imagery Exercises, Shizuto Masunaga, Japan Publications, Tokyo, 1979.

Barefoot Shiatsu, Shizuko Yamamoto, Japan Publications, Tokyo, 1979.

Do It Yourself Shiatsu, Waturu Ohashi, Allan & Unwin, London, 1977.

Tsubo, Katsusuke Serizawa, Japan Publications, Tokyo, 1985.

Shiatsu and Stretching, Toru Namikoshi, Japan Publications, Tokyo, 1985.

How To See Your Health: Book of Oriental Diagnosis, Michio Kushi, Japan Publications, Tokyo, 1980.

Macrobiotics and Human Behaviour, William Tara, Japan Publications, Tokyo, 1984.

Acupuncture Medicine, Yoshiaki Omura, Japan Publications, Tokyo, 1982.

The Yellow Emperor's Classic of Internal Medicine, Ilza Veith, Berkeley, Los Angeles, London – University of California Press, 1966.

Chinese Medicine, Ted J. Kaptchuk, Rider, London, 1983.

Awaken Healing Energy Through the Tao, Mantak Chia, Aurora Press, New York, 1983.

Zen Mind, Beginner's Mind, Shunryu Suzuki, Weatherhill, New York, 1970.

Tao Teh Ching, Lao Tzu, Frederick Ungar Publishing, London – Wildwood House Ltd, 1958.

INDEX

Numbers in *italic* refer to illustrations

sexual libido, 10, 58, 79
sharp voice, 51
shen cycles, 66–68, *67*
shiatsu: after effects, 87; case
    histories, 78–81; differs from
    acupuncture, 13; differs from
    massage, 13–14; doctor's
    advice, 16–17; effective help,
    i; effects of, 5–6; helps
    conditions, 6; history of, 3–4;
    how it helps, 4–5; influence
    of life energy, 12, *12*;
    lifeforce, 11; maintains good
    health, 14–16; people who are
    unsuitable for, 16; specific
    conditions helped by, 72–81;
    treatment, 82–89; what it is,
    1; *see also* treatment
shoshin, 46
shoulder tension, 78–79
shoulders, 54–55, 77
sing-song voice, 51
skeletal system, 7
skin, 6–7
skin: condition, 50; eruptions,
    10, 29, 30; texture, 48; tone,
    85
sleep, 103
smoking, 72
soil, 71
spinal injuries, 82
spinal problems, 17
spinal vertebrae, 77
spine, 77
spiritual conditions controlled
    by viscera, 27
spiritual hunger, 10
spleen, 33, 54
sports injuries, 16, 76
spring, 64–65
stamina, 14
stiffness, 5, 28
stomach, 33
stomach, avoid a full, 85
stomach meridian energy, 10
stress, 5, 11, 12, 14
stress, exercises to relieve, 92–94
stress-related illness, 82
stress-related symptoms, 52
stretching, 3, 5, 94–98, *94–97*

stroke, 14
structural disorders, 77
sugar, 88
summer, 65
surgery, 17, 50
swimming, 91
'switch', 42
sympathetic systems, 12
symptoms, 47
symptoms, energy movement,
    30–32
symptoms, energy relationships,
    32–37
symptoms, separate, 5

tai chi, 2, 90
tan den, 93
tao, 23
telepathy, 12
tennis, 91
tension, 5, 54
thigh, 58
thumb, 1, 55
toes, 60
tongue diagnosis, 60–61, *61*
torso, 55, *57*
touch, i, 1
touch diagnosis, 50, 83
toxic elimination, 5
toxins, 62, 75
transformations table, 70–71
treatment: cost of, 89;
    self-treatment, 88–89; how
    many needed, 84; what it
    involves, 82–89
triple heater, 35
tsubo, 2–3, 14, 28, 29, 44, 85
tumour, 53
twelve principles of nature, 23

ulcers, 41
urination, 75

vase (*tsubo*), 28
vegetables, 21
viscera, 27
visual diagnosis, 47–48, 83
vital organs, 18
voice, 51

MORE BOOKS FROM OPTIMA

ALTERNATIVE HEALTH SERIES

This series is designed to provide factual information and
practical advice about alternative therapies. While
including essential details of theory and history, the books
concentrate on what patients can expect during
treatment, how they should prepare for it, what questions
will be asked and why, what form the treatment will take,
and what it will 'feel' like and how soon they can expect to
respond.

ACUPUNCTURE by Dr Michael Nightingale
Acupuncture is a traditional Chinese therapy which
usually (but not always) uses needles to stimulate the
body's own energy and so bring healing.
ISBN 0 356 12426 6
Price (in UK only) **£3.95**

ALEXANDER TECHNIQUE by Chris Stevens
Alexander Technique is a way of becoming more aware of
balance, posture and movement in everyday activities. It
can not only cure various complaints related to posture,
such as backache, but teaches people to use their body
more effectively and reduces stress.
ISBN 0 356 12430 4
Price (in UK only) **£4.99**

AROMATHERAPY by Gill Martin
Aromatherapy uses the essential oils of plants, which are
massaged into the skin, added to baths or taken internally
to treat a variety of ailments and enhance general
well-being.
ISBN 0 356 17113 2
Price (in UK only) **£4.99**

CHIROPRACTIC by Susan Moore
Chiropractic is based on the belief that disease is caused
by the misalignment of the bones in the spine.
Chiropractors heal by manipulating the spine gently back
into its correct position.
ISBN 0 356 12433 9
Price (in UK only) **£3.95**

HERBAL MEDICINE by Anne McIntyre
Herbal medicine has been known for thousands of years.
It is an entirely natural system of medicine which relies on
the therapeutic quality of plants to enhance the body's
recuperative powers, and so bring health – without any
undesirable side effects.
ISBN 0 356 12429 0
Price (in UK only) **£3.95**

HOMEOPATHY by Dr Nelson Brunton
Homeopathy is based on the principle, discovered by
Samuel Hahnemann some 200 years ago, that like cures
like. In this system of medicine, diseases are treated with
very small quantities of herbs, minerals or drugs.
ISBN 0 356 12427 4
Price (in UK only) **£4.99**

HYPNOSIS by Ursula Markham
Hypnosis has a remarkable record of curing a wide range
of ills. Ursula Markham a practising hypnotherapist,
explains how, by releasing inner tensions, hypnosis can
help people to heal themselves.
ISBN 0 356 12432 0
Price (in UK only) **£3.95**

MEDITATION by Erica Smith and Nicholas Wilks
Meditation is a state of inner stillness which has been
cultivated by mystics for thousands of years. The main
reason for its recent popularity is that regular practice has
been found to improve mental and physical health, largely
due to its role in alleviating stress.
ISBN 0 356 14569 7
Price (in UK only) **£4.99**

OSTEOPATHY by Stephen Sandler
Osteopathy started in the USA in the 1870s, and has since
spread to many other countries. It is a manipulative
therapy, in which the osteopath heals by adjusting the
position of bones and tissues.
ISBN 0 356 12428 2
Price (in UK only) **£3.95**

All Optima books are available at your bookshop or newsagent, or can be ordered from the following address:

Optima, Cash Sales Department,
PO Box 11, Falmouth, Cornwall TR10 9EN

Please send cheque or postal order (no currency), and allow 60p for postage and packing for the first book, plus 25p for the second book and 15p for each additional book ordered up to a maximum charge of £1.90 in the UK.

Customers in Eire and BFPO please allow 60p for the first book, 25p for the second book plus 15p per copy for the next 7 books, thereafter 9p per book.

Overseas customers please allow £1.25 for postage and packing for the first book and 28p per copy for each additional book.